Series in Ethnicity, Medicine, and Psychoanalysis   VOLUME 3

Clinical Stories and

Their Translations

Series in Ethnicity, Medicine, and Psychoanalysis   VOLUME 3

Clinical Stories
and
Their Translations

HOWARD F. STEIN
and MAURICE APPREY

University Press of Virginia

Charlottesville and London

THE UNIVERSITY PRESS OF VIRGINIA
Copyright © 1990 by the Rector and Visitors
of the University of Virginia

First published 1990

Library of Congress Cataloging-in-Publication Data
  Clinical stories and their translations / Howard F. Stein and
Maurice Apprey.
    p. cm. — (Series in ethnicity, medicine, and psychoanalysis : v. 3)
    Includes bibliographies and index.
    ISBN 0-8139-1241-5
    1. Medical history taking—Psychological aspects. 2. Physician and
patient. 3. Sick—Family relationships. 4. Medical care—
Psychological aspects. 5. Psychoanalytic interpretation. I. Apprey,
Maurice, 1947–   . II. Title. III. Series.
    [DNLM: 1. Ethnopsychology. 2. Family Practice. 3. Physician-
Patient Relations. 4. Psychoanalytic Interpretation. 5. Psychoanalytic
Therapy. WM 460.7 S819c]
RC65.S74 1990
616.07′51—dc20
DNLM/DLC
for Library of Congress   89-16615
                                                                      CIP

Printed in the United States of America

Dedicated to

Vamık D. Volkan, M.D.

Friend, colleague, mentor

Contents

Foreword

G. GAYLE STEPHENS, M.D.

It requires temerity to write a serious book of clinical stories for medical educational purposes nowadays, but it takes audacity to write them in a patois of psychoanalysis and anthropology. The authors of this volume seem not at all intimidated that anecdotes, even interesting ones, have all but disappeared from the pages of the most reputable modern medical publications; or that psychoanalysis has been obsolete within mainstream medicine for at least a couple of decades.

On the contrary, they insist that a good deal of the most important clinical work with ordinary patients lies precisely in the capacity of physicians (and other health professionals) to appreciate the clinical relevance of how patients come to understand their own lives; not only their lives as patients within the medical care system, but also their membership in particular families, social classes, geographical regions, and belief systems. Moreover, the authors also believe that physicians' understanding of their own experiences as members of these same groups is an important variable in their capacity to be therapeutic with their patients.

What is required between clinicians and patients is a coherent, convincing, and shared account of how things came to be as they are, and what might be done to ameliorate the debilitating effects of disease or injury, self-defeating behavior, destructive intimate relationships, and ineffective treatment. Such an account is not easily come by. It is part discovery and part invention, in which facts are given meaning and linked to each other in ways that are at the same time personal and universal. Such a creative account cannot be imposed through superior wisdom and knowledge; it emerges within a real relationship between clinician and patient, one that is safe and nonexploitive, wherein each party is at various times leader and follower. Since the relationship is real, it is not wholly rational and objective, not merely expert-client or authoritarian; it is more like participant observation, what the authors refer to as ethnographic. It takes into account data that seem nonrational, irrational, or even absurd.

While this methodology may appear daunting to the novice, unattractive to the technologist, or hopeless to the organ-system expert, it is the best and most therapeutic approach to certain types of clinical problems and the patients who embody them. Each patient-care experience can be conducted as a piece of clinical research, observing, imagining, and testing hypotheses. Compared with other methods, the ethnographic experiment more openly presumes that the researcher is a variable, a fact often obscured in research of other types. Each patient is a "series of one" in which the process of diagnosis, i.e., understanding the story, is also the treatment. What is truly therapeutic is more likely to be valid, although the authors carefully point out that not all "healing" is truly therapeutic.

What we have in this book is a number of such experiments. With one exception (chapter 3), the patients are not extraordinary. They are drawn from family practice settings and psychiatric practice. Their problems are familiar to all generalist physicians: an anorexic girl in a chaotic family, a woman with a spinal-cord injury, a disabled veteran, an infant who failed to thrive, a farmer who postponed medical treatment, cigarette addiction, emotional difficulties in school. What the authors bring to bear on these problems and patients are a method and a theory. The method is ethno-graphic—i.e., participant observation; the theory is a particular view of psychoanalysis, especially its topographic model and its understanding of projective identification.

The outcomes of this process for the patients are not quick and easy cures, but a chance to participate with their clinicians in the reconstruction of the meaning of their critical life experiences that led to or perpetuated their illnesses. They are empowered to revise their self-understanding of what happened to them, and what keeps happening, by means of a new translation of explanations that is more rational, more comprehensive, and truer to their facts. They become able to make stepwise changes in their behavior away from the unexamined and repetitious dramas that perpetuate their illnesses. This is liberation and therapy. It should be emphasized that patients are not expected merely to substitute the physician's explanations for their own— which might not be therapeutic at all, especially if the physicians have not reconstructed their own stories—but to test the mutually developed new translations in the crucible of their lives.

What are the authors' warrants for appealing to ethnography and re-habilitating psychoanalysis as a combined clinical method at a time when mainstream medicine, including psychiatry, is still preoccupied with tech-nological cure of the body as a protoplasmic machine? What need is there to focus on the subjectivity of the patient when the primary ethos of modern medicine has been to cleanse itself from the messiness of intimate personal relationships in favor of the purer science of objectivity and detachment?

In the first place, all practitioners of medicine are inundated with patients who either have not benefited from mainstream medicine or have been made worse by it. There are casualties from high-tech medicine who need some-

thing other than reprocessing through that system at enormous cost. Main-stream medicine is short on conversation, even shorter on genuine dialog. The bulk of modern medical care is given by strangers who barely know their patients' names. Moreover, since the rejection of psychoanalysis, after its academic apogee in the 1950s, no new medical psychology has emerged. We have a number of psychologies, but none has achieved orthodox status. Behaviorism, educational psychology, developmental psychology, and family therapy have their advocates, alongside a number of pop psychologies and quasi-religious psychologies; but none of these have natural ties to medicine and none are taught in a rigorous, systematic way to physicians.

Perhaps it is time to reconsider what a modernized psychoanalysis could offer medicine. Paradoxically, psychoanalysis never disappeared from the arts—novels, plays, painting—or even from history. New fields of history that utilize psychoanalytic ideas have emerged in the past twenty years—psychohistory, the history of childhood, and cultural history as interpreted by such Freudian historians as Peter Gay. It is only in medicine that the rejection appears to have been nearly complete, and perhaps there are good reasons for that. The clinical method of traditional psychoanalysis, tedious, time-consuming, and interminable, was never adapted to the realities of physicians' work schedules. Its language, much of it derived from classical mythology, was strange and unpalatable, and training in it was inaccessible. The whole psychoanalytic enterprise seemed shrouded in mystery and secrecy, unlike the more public manner in which other fields of medical research were conducted. Psychoanalysis was never verifiable nor falsifiable by the same standards that applied to other medical sciences, so that even though it gained a good deal of academic power in major departments of psychiatry in the 1950s, it was unable to hold its ground and finally had to retreat to the safety of its institutes outside the mainstream of academic medicine.

The authors have not addressed all these problems, but in the ethno-graphic method they create the possibility for a psychoanalytically informed physician to apply this knowledge to the routines of daily clinical work. Ethnography, as explained by Stein (chapter 1), requires a genuine relation-ship between doctor and patient in which both are trying to understand and find a solution to the patient's clinical problems. It sees both doctor and patient within the context of their real lives, and allows everything that happens between them to become grist for the mill of mutual understanding. It requires no couch, is much more flexible about the ritualized rules of behavior, and uses no foreign languages or literary metaphors. Ethnography might do for psychoanalysis what Wittgenstein and others did for meta-physics, namely, convert its mysteries to the meaning of ordinary language.

It remains to be seen whether these authors have advanced the cause of personal medicine, but it appears that they are working on the problem in a creative way. These stories about real patients and real doctors do not strain our credulity, and they offer readers the hope that they, too, might come to understand their patients and themselves better. That is bound to be therapeutic. One way or another, doctors will continue to have to deal with the nonrational, irrational, and absurd aspects of human behavior. If ethnography and psychoanalysis are not the right means to do this, we must continue to search for better alternatives, but this book is a cogent defense of that pair.

Preface

This book is about the stories that patients and clinicians of all professions compose and tell, and the influence of these stories upon the clinical encounter and work. In clinical stories—the clinician's, the patient's, and that common one negotiated between them—there is usually more than is obviously manifest. Indeed, it is most therapeutic when clinician and patient alike are able to explore the relationship between the presenting story (the manifest picture, so to speak) and the underlying, mostly hidden story (the unconscious picture, so to speak). Since it is the professional responsibility of the clinician to help the patient (and not vice versa), then it becomes the responsibility of the clinician to be able to tolerate those underlying stories in himself or herself in order to help the patient gain access to his or her own. This ideal is, of course, far from accepted in most medical, therapy, and counseling training. Implicitly, much of medical and generically clinical education consists of offering initiate-trainees those *translations* of patients' or clients' stories that will validate their own defensive organization—translations that take the form of official theories, methods, procedures, and knowledge itself. This book is about the stories that practitioners of all disciplines construct, and about the process and problem of translation that often interferes with clinicians' ability to elicit their patients' and clients' latent stories.

A fruitful approach to understanding physicians' and other clinicians' clinical accounts or stories derives from the psychoanalytical topographic model that is hierarchically organized into unconscious, preconscious, and conscious aspects of thought, feeling, and action. This dynamic model of mental process helps us to understand and teach about physicians' (and other practitioners') unrecognized responses to patients (technically termed countertransference), and thereby to entertain the possibility that there exists an implicit story beneath the official, explicit one. It addresses the relationship between formal clinical knowledge structures (e.g., official diagnostic criteria, decision trees, and treatment protocols) and the actual process clinicians go through in constructing etiological accounts, diagnostic interpretations, treatment plans, and outcome evaluations. This model likewise helps us to entertain the possibility that seemingly rational, scientific, "official" clinical models have some irrational aspect or can bear the burden of (be used for) unconscious purposes.

In recent years there has been considerable interest in the formal logic of biomedical decision making (Cebul and Beck 1985; Weinstein et al. 1980). At the same time there has been renewed interest in the personal, more subjective aspects of clinical thinking and decision making. Several authors have highlighted the role of countertransference (Balint 1957; Katz 1984; Ross and Phipps 1986; Smith 1984, 1985, 1986; Stein 1982, 1983, 1985, 1986; Stein and Apprey 1985), and related family-of-origin issues (Christie-Seely et al 1984; Crouch 1986; Mengel 1985, 1987), as a major determinant of these more subjective dimensions of clinical performance. Because the formal logic of clinical thinking is frequently opposed by this subjective dimension (Smith 1984, 1986), it is important to develop a framework within which to better understand and teach about this conflict between the formal and subjective dimensions of clinical decision making. (We hasten to add that a physician could also appropriate the biomedical model or formal reasoning for unconscious purposes.) One could speak of three intertwined medical domains in biomedicine: (1) The prescriptive, formal logic of clinical decision making, (2) interviewing skills and techniques, and (3) unconscious or countertransference issues. All three are aspects of the structure and function of the mental organization of the clinicians who are engaged in clinical decision making. Moreover, formal decision making and interviewing are closely related constructs and processes.

Sigmund Freud's (1905, 1923) topographical or hierarchical model of the mind is a valuable tool for understanding these three medical domains. It tells us that physicians' mental operations are governed by conscious, preconscious, and unconscious influences. According to this model, formal algorithms, decision trees, and learned interviewing skills are primarily functions of the physician's conscious and preconscious; i.e., they are mostly within one's conscious perceptual awareness or can be easily summoned into consciousness for decision making. Much of the content and function of this mental operation can be characterized as "secondary process," rational, and reality based.

Nevertheless, because conscious and preconscious mechanisms are strongly influenced by the unconscious, supposedly rational clinical thinking and interviewing may be considerably altered by unconscious processes and can, in fact, be governed by the unconscious. These unconscious responses can determine the physician's behavior with the patient. Such unrecognized feelings and behaviors are the same ones that produce problems with "difficult" patients and that lead to ineffective physician-patient interactions in many other circumstances. This occurs because these deeply ingrained feelings override more recently acquired, rational information (about decision making and interviewing) when it is in conflict with them.

The importance of unrecognized responses toward patients is that they can produce harm to the patient, missed diagnoses, improper treatment, poor practitioner-patient interactions, and mutual dissatisfaction. That such responses are nearly universal only magnifies their significance and the educational need to address them. Formal models are ideal and prescriptive; they specify how physicians or other clinicians ought to think. Formal models are also abstract, impersonal, and bureaucratic artifacts; actual clinical decision making is situational and personal. Countertransference responses result in clinicians' assessments of patients that are not based entirely upon the reality of patients' situations, but, rather, upon clinicians' personal, unrecognized responses. Countertransference thus may interfere with the desired patient-centered focus and lead inadvertently to a practitioner-centered approach. The topographical model provides a format for understanding and teaching this concept. (The preceding four paragraphs are adapted from Smith and Stein 1987).

Complicating the process of eliciting deeper stories and of moving "vertically" between levels (in the sense of unconscious, preconscious, and conscious levels), is the fact that hierarchically and developmentally speaking, these levels do not speak the same language. There is thus not only a frequent "confusion of tongues" (Ferenczi 1933) between the adult's and child's perception of the world but also an often insurmountable problem of "translating" both between clinician and adult patient's ostensible or manifest language and between the various levels within oneself as well. Calogeras succinctly writes, for instance, that

> Our accumulated analytic evidence [on the nature of recall of childhood phenomena] suggests that there is no such thing as a pure (or undistorted) recall of a child experience; rather in the recovery of an early childhood memory we are confronted not with the recall of something repressed in the usual sense of the term, but with a synthesizing and creative act in which something can for the first time be understood and put into secondary process language. As a consequence, the conclu-

sion follows that such a recalled traumatic experience has never been
put into secondary process terms because the original experience had
taken place at a level of ego-integration and during a stage of development which did not make it available at that time for preconscious or
conscious integration in the ego (1982:484–85).

For instance, many people "remember" only through actions or
deeds (acting out) or physically felt symptoms, and not through
feeling and verbalizing; indeed, the action is a repetition compulsion and compromise, the purpose of which is to prevent dangerous
and frightening thoughts and feelings from becoming conscious.
Making further elusive the *completeness* of the patient's and clinician's story—and therefore what the clinician can tolerate to hear
and respond to in the patient—is the fact that both reality (outer)
and fantasy (inner) must be taken into account. Masterson recently
writes that "The clinical evidence is overwhelming that *both* what
happened—reality—and the patient's later intrapsychic elabora-
tions of it—fantasy—matter a great deal" (1985:170).

For patients and clinicians of all types (physicians, psychiatrists,
psychoanalysts, clinical psychologists, family therapists, social
workers, pastoral counselors, medical behavioral scientists), together with their families, communities, and cultures, clinical work
is the construction and interpretation of stories. This book is thus
addressed to those health professionals and behavioral scientists
interested in better understanding, eliciting, interpreting, and
working within patients' stories—and their own as well.

If the clinical "story behind the story"—to borrow a phrase from
journalism—is the central *substantive* theme of this volume, then its
companion central *methodological* theme is the utility of integrating
the psychoanalytic and ethnographic methods of inquiry as a means
of eliciting or gaining access to this story. To label the method used
as either psychoanalytically oriented applied ethnography or ethnographically oriented psychoanalysis is subtly to perpetuate the
false dichotomy identified as the spurious split between "culture"
and "personality" (Spiro 1951) or group and individual. Almost
four decades ago Spiro noted that "the development of personality
and the acquisition of culture are one and the same process" (ibid.
31) and that "the culture of any individual is incorporated within his
personality" (ibid. 43) even as much of culture is projected and
experienced consciously as "existing" outside the self. At their best,
ethnographically sensitive psychoanalysis and psychoanalytically
sensitive applied ethnography have an identical goal, whether the
"object" is an individual, a family, or a group: the depths of feelings,

meanings, symbols, fantasies, myths, and rituals that organize that person, family, or group. Whether it be called psychoanalytic ethnography or ethnographic psychoanalysis, it consists of a way of thinking about, systematically gathering, and utilizing in various problem-solving situations human stories.

Now, superficially, several seemingly major differences can be noted—but quickly dispensed with. One is that according to the classical practice of psychoanalysis, the analysand or patient lies supine on a couch, with the analyst out of view, seated in a chair at the head of the couch; on the other hand, the ethnographic fieldworker works and lives in the thick of things, so to speak, through naturalistic and participant observation and open-ended interviewing in the informant's home, community, or culture. A second dichotomy is that while the analytic patient comes to the analyst or psychiatrist for change (offering powerful resistance to change in the process), the ethnographer goes to the field only to observe, never to intrude or change the informant or native.

However, even in "pure" ethnographic fieldwork—such as was initiated by anthropologist Bronislaw Malinowski in the Trobriand Islands (off northern New Guinea) during the First World War— the very presence of the observer, together with the observer's avowed interests, introduces subtle change in those under observation. Many psychoanalysts and psychoanalytically oriented psychotherapists now attempt to familiarize themselves thoroughly with the patient's family and wider social circumstances (e.g., Devereux 1951; Spiegel 1971). Both in process and product, competent clinical psychoanalysis *is* fieldwork, and insightful ethnography *is* a clinical (therapeutic) experience. Although pure anthropological researchers strive to avoid imposing external value judgments upon, or serving as agents of culture change in, the communities in which they work, applied anthropologists—such as are employed as clinical teachers and supervisors, urban and international development consultants, and minority-group language-education specialists—are called upon to help foster change, or at least to provide information to policymakers about the conditions that foster and impede such change.

Yet, even the distinction between "pure" and "applied" anthropology should not be too sharply drawn with respect to the action, interaction, and psychodynamics in fieldwork. For as the psychologically sensitive ethnographer elicits and listens to the informant's or community member's story, he or she helps the informant to tell it. The story thus told will inevitably be more conscious, more complete, than the "native" account prior to the intervention with the ethnographer. In pure or applied ethnography, as in psychoanalytic therapy, the informant's or patient's story is the product of a largely *playful* interaction. Even in pure ethnography, both ethnographer and informant are often profoundly changed by the encounter. Viewed psychodynamically, the *kinds* of resistances patients offer psychoanalysts in the consulting room (protecting themselves against painful insights and feelings that would constitute the story behind the story) are no different from the kinds of protective armor in which individuals, families, communities, agencies, and nations cloak themselves toward various change agents whom they employ to help them change.

For the astute psychoanalyst and applied ethnographer alike, understanding a system is inherent in the process of intervening in it. Such understanding is not *prior to* the intervention; it is never outside of it. Moreover, for both, such a process of understanding is simultaneously a voyage of self-understanding *and* a collaborative effort with the patient, informant, colleague, or agency.

In this book, the coauthors, a psychoanalytic/medical anthropologist (Stein) and a child analyst (Apprey) demonstrate the wide application of the psychoanalytic-ethnographic method in ordinary *clinical practice,* in *clinical teaching,* and in *clinical supervision.* In sum, the authors' main themes are (1) the immense depth and breadth of clinical stories, (2) the psychoanalytic-ethnographic method as a means of gaining access to them, and (3) the need for clinicians of all specialties to become conversant with both the stories and the method for uncovering them. This book thus offers a clinical mode of inquiry that will deepen and widen clinical knowledge, practice, teaching, and supervision. It proposes a method with which clinicians can explore—together with their patients, students, colleagues, and apprentices—the depth and breadth of meaning that is intrinsic to stories of health, sickness, and healing.

REFERENCES

Balint, M. 1957. *The doctor, his patient, and the illness.* New York: International Universities Press.

Calogeras, Roy C. 1982. Sleepwalking and the traumatic experience. *International Journal of Psychoanalysis* 63:483–89.

Cebul, R. D., and L. H. Beck. 1985. *Teaching medical decision making.* New York: Praeger Special Studies.

Christie-Seely, J., R. Fernandez, G. Paradis, Y. Talbot, and R. Turcotte. 1984. The physician's family. In *Working with the family in primary care: A systems approach to health and illness,* edited by J. Christie-Seely, 524–46. New York: Praeger.

Crouch, M. 1986. Working with one's own family: Another path for professional development. *Family Medicine* 18:93–98.

Devereux, G. 1951. *Reality and dream: The psychotherapy of a Plains Indian.* New York: International Universities Press.

Ferenczi, S. 1933. Confusion of tongues between adults and the child. *International Journal of Psycho-Analysis* 30:225–30.

Freud, S. 1905. Jokes and their relation to the unconscious. In *The standard edition of the complete psychological works of Sigmund Freud (SE)* 8, translated by J. Strachey, 3–236 (especially p. 164). London: Hogarth Press, 1960.

———. 1923. The ego and the id. *SE* 19, translated by J. Strachey, 3–66 (especially pp. 13–18). London: Hogarth Press, 1961.

Katz, J. 1984. *The silent world of doctor and patient.* New York: The Free Press/ Macmillan.

Masterson, J. F. 1985. *The real self.* New York: Brunner/Mazel.

Mengel, M. B. 1985. Collaboration with family therapists: Dealing with physician's family of origin issues. *Working Together* 1:10–11.

———. 1987. Physician ineffectiveness due to family-of-origin issues. *Family Systems Medicine* 5(2):176–90.

Ross, J. L., and E. Phipps. 1986. Physician-patient power struggles: Their role in noncompliance. *Family Medicine* 18:99–101.

Smith, R. C. 1984. Teaching interviewing skills to medical students: The issue of "countertransference." *Journal of Medical Education* 59:582–88.

———. 1985. A clinical approach to the somatizing patient. *The Journal of Family Practice* 21:294–301.

———. 1986. Unrecognized responses and feelings of residents and fellows during interviews of patients. *Journal of Medical Education* 61:982–84.

Smith, R. C., and H. F. Stein. 1987. A topographical model of clinical decision making and interviewing. *Family Medicine* 19(5):361–63.

Spiegel, J. 1971. *Transactions: The interplay between individual, family, and society.* New York: Science House.

Spiro, M. E. 1951. Culture and personality: The natural history of a false dichotomy. *Psychiatry* 14:19–46.

Stein, H. F. 1982. Physician-patient transaction through the analysis of countertransference: A study in role relationship and unconscious meaning. *Medical Anthropology* 6:165–82.

———. 1983. The influence of countertransference upon the clinical relationship and decision-making. *Continuing Education for the Family Physician* 18:625–30.

———. 1985. *The psychodynamics of medical practice: Unconscious factors in patient care.* Berkeley/Los Angeles: University of California Press.

———. 1986. "Sick people" and "trolls": A contribution to the understanding of the dynamics of physician explanatory models. *Culture, Medicine and Psychiatry* 10:221–29.

Stein, H. F., and M. Apprey. 1985. *Context and dynamics in clinical knowledge,* vol. 1 of the Series in Ethnicity, Medicine, and Psychoanalysis. Charlottesville: University Press of Virginia.

Weinstein, M. C., H. V. Fineberg, A. S. Elstein, H. S. Frazier, D. Neuhauser,

R. R. Neutra, and B. J. McNeil. 1980. *Clinical decision analysis.* Philadelphia, Pa.: W. B. Saunders Co.

ACKNOWLEDGMENTS

Gratitude is expressed to the University Press of Virginia for its continued and vigorous support for this series in Ethnicity, Medicine, and Psychoanalysis. We wish to thank Vamık D. Volkan, M.D., for his personal and professional support in the preparation of this volume. To G. Gayle Stephens, M.D., goes a great debt of gratitude for inviting the original version of "What Is Therapeutic in Clinical Relationships?" presented at the Advanced Forum in Family Medicine, Keystone, Colorado, 28 September 1984. Margaret A. Stein, M.A., diligently typed, edited, and proofread much of this book, as she did with the previous volumes in this series.

COPYRIGHT NOTE

Clinical Stories and
Their Translations

Introduction

HOWARD F. STEIN AND MAURICE APPREY

We know more than can be formulated in one finite systematized
scheme of abstractions, however important that scheme may be
in the elucidation of some aspect of the order of things
(Whitehead 1960:137)

All clinical work and clinical education—indeed, all human communication—rests upon the attempt to make emotionally compatible sense out of experience. Treatment plans, theories, religions,
political movements, are all efforts to construct *stories* (narratives or
discourses, in social science terminology) that create and impose
coherence and meaning on the inner and outer worlds alike. Now,
in this book that discusses those "stories" that doctors and patients
tell, hear, and compose, our use of the term *story* differs considerably from some conventional connotations of the word. In one
popular use, *story* refers to such diverse meanings as fiction (as
contrasted with fact, objectivity, or reality), the work of the childlike
or poetic imagination (as contrasted with accounts by scientists or
physicians), even lying (i.e., telling a story versus telling the truth).

There is yet another popular use of the word *story*, one quite in
keeping with our own usage throughout this volume. In this popular usage, such a story is often a true story, an historical account, as
in the etymology of the word, *historia*. Moreover, one often refers to
the difficulty of getting to the bottom of a story. In the field of
broadcast journalism, for instance, a newscaster might begin with
"There was a story out of Chicago today, . . ." and momentarily
follow it up with "And now for the story behind the story. . . ." From
the viewpoint of depth psychology, the story consists of the whole
story, the beginning, the end (the underlying story or stories), and
the process of getting there, thus including the telling of the story
and the implied relationship in the narration.

In this work, *story* refers to the process and structure of any
account, whether this be to oneself, between clinician and patient, a
shared organization of ideas within an institution (say, a hospital or
medical department), or common to an entire culture. Our interest
here is in how clinicians and patients, families and medical staffs,

put their clinical stories together. Official, often conventional, standardized, and stylized stories about how things *ought* to go together (e.g., diagnosis of disease, treatment decision trees, patient compliance with medical advice) may differ markedly from how those stories actually turn out (i.e., what social scientists often describe as the dichotomy between the ideal and the real). We will examine further what stories clinicians and patients compose to account for this turn of events.

The aesthetic intent and effect of telling stories is to convey completeness and to validate their tellers' sensibility about what is true. This is often achieved by *filling in the blanks,* so to speak, with details and assumptions that make the sequence and outcome coherent. Patients, families, and clinical decision makers, it turns out, have as many "story lines" as do novels, movies, and television soap operas (cf. Kris on "personal myth" [1956], Ferreira on "family myth" [1963], and Stierlin on "group fantasy" [1973]). What is more, cognitive-emotional lapses or loopholes in official story lines (whether they be theological, philosophical, medical, or political) are filled in and supplemented by subsidiary stories or themes that people create in order to make the story more satisfactory (see Spiro 1982). Even widely shared stories are never totally static: the "folk" versions are always adding to the "high culture" authorized versions, occasionally producing outright revolutions that lead to the establishment of a new "folk" tale as the Official Truth (e.g., the Russian Revolution, the Protestant Reformation). In both cases, expectations as to how ideas (and their associated feelings) ought to hang together lead to orthodoxies of belief and ritual alike for all institutions from medicine to religion; the opposite side of this is heresy or apostasy: the way ideas should and must *not* be put together.

To place all this in the clinical context, we might raise the following questions: What stories are clinicians and clinical teachers trying to hear and to teach? What stories do we need—can we bear—to hear and to tell? What stories are patients, families, colleagues, residents trying to tell us or to hear from us; and what are they trying to avoid telling us or hearing from us as well? Such questions bring us to the doorstep of inquiring into the mental and interpersonal and cultural or group *function* of these stories. Akin to myths and fairy tales universally, the internal and interpersonal function of stories is to diminish anxiety and guilt and to help give coherence to the self (Boyer 1979). They do so, however, at the cost of deeper knowledge of the self, interruption of repetitions of past trauma, and greater knowledge of reality. Instead of reality, it is the story itself that must continually be reaffirmed—ironic and especially dangerous when the enterprise is labeled scientific. In clinician-patient interactions, often diagnosis and treatment consist of formulating what might be called replacement stories (akin to secondary revision following dreams) that prevent the disturbing deeper stories from surfacing.

Culturally conventionalizing stories, as well as dyadic ones (e.g., doctor-patient), take what is disturbingly personal and turn it into what is reassuringly impersonal—for doctor, patient, family, staff, and society alike. Medical histories and physicals, diagnoses, technical procedures, case reports, decision trees, and the like become formulistic and stereotypic clinical genres. As in religious rite, participants, made to feel better by the story held in common, harbor an at least implicit consensus that no other story is acceptable, and that only certain kinds of "data" are acceptable for inclusion in the story (e.g., "hard," biomedical laboratory reports versus "soft," psychosocial information obtained through home visit or psychotherapy). Patients are treated and students and residents are trained largely to validate and pass on the culturally favorite and most reassuring stories (theories, models, treatment protocols) that sustain participants' defensive organization and their relationships with one another.

The practice of and training for scientific medicine and the various psycho- and family-therapies is often unwittingly undermined or sabotaged by practitioners and educators who employ various theories, skills, and procedures for largely defensive purposes. Instead of fostering greater access to the patient's many levels of stories (from unconscious to conscious) by fostering such access within the clinician, much of clinical education and practice instead fosters the *translation of the patient's story into that story compatible with and reaffirming of the therapist's defensive organization*—and that of the institution or profession the clinician represents. Thus, unwittingly, clinicians unconsciously shore up their own identity— and reaffirm the verity of their own stories—*through* patient care. Diagnosis and treatment—patient care—far from being the ends, are in fact to a considerable degree means to ends of which the clinician is largely unaware.

How can one truly listen and respond to another when one cannot afford—and has never been trained—NOT to translate the patient's world back into a comfortable clinical one? How can what is genuinely therapeutic occur when the story that must be recounted is the one that neither patient nor therapist nor teacher nor institution-writ-large can tolerate to hear? In all societies, people *translate* vexing, painful, unconscious stories into cozening conscious tales that keep the underlying hurts and conflicts unresolved by searching for further symbolic and ritual solutions. The same is true for most clinical training and practice. This book is about the necessity of overcoming that penchant to translation, and the difficulty in doing so.

Simon Grolnick writes that "We understand each other by understanding ourselves, and vice versa. A reflection on the understanding of 'the other' helps to bring about self-understanding. (Winnicott maintained that we help our patient most in working out the effect of our mistakes on them.) In other words, a misunderstanding of the object helps the subject to know himself. Both subject (and subjectivity) and object (and objectivity) are involved: paradoxically, they are inseparable" (1987:138). Stated differently, for researcher and clinician alike, knowledge of our own stories helps us to elicit and to listen to the depth of others' stories. As we experience, tolerate, and come to understand our own anxiety evoked *as* we listen to their stories, we can better understand our own—which in turn gives us greater access to theirs, and so on.

Peoples' "stories of sickness" (Brody 1987) or illness narratives are embodied both in their accounts of themselves when they fall ill and in their responses to others. This holds for laity, medical practitioners, psychotherapists, family therapists, and folk healers alike. In a book that explores literary works that deal with sickness, Brody eloquently writes that "just as to be sick is to sense an unpleasant disruption of the self-body unity ('ontological assault') . . . , to perceive sickness or disability in others is to be reminded of one's own vulnerability and mortality in an equally unpleasant and threatening way. Thus much reaction to sickness that superficially appears to be solely outward-directed (that is, toward meeting the needs of the sick person) is in reality also inner-directed as an attempt to remove, resolve, or transcend this inner threat to integrity" (1987:110). In most official clinical—not only biomedical—renderings, from textbooks to case conferences and medical records, what Brody has just described is rarely regarded or recorded as part of "the case." To evince countertransference (subjectivity) is to be unprofessional; it is banished from awareness. Indeed, as we shall illustrate amply throughout this volume, much of clinical theory, method, protocols, and the like are used, if not "designed," to serve as collective defenses against the recognition and feeling that the clinician has much in common with the patient.

In biomedicine, one of the most formidable bulwarks against this blurring of boundaries, is the conviction, if not the myth, that medicine is to be equated with science—as in the term *medical science*. Yet Munson (1981) has recently argued that medical practice, while using and advancing science, cannot itself be logically construed to be science. While science (at least ideally) seeks to discover truth and measures success by such discovery, medicine seeks new knowledge in order to cure patients, and physicians have (or at least espouse) a fiduciary responsibility to their patients.

Clinical research and "basic science" are, of course, socially linked in that they are delegated the cultural mission of finding the causes of disease and their treatments. By borrowing theory, method, and authority from science, medicine—and other clinical specialties as well—can construct stories of patients' afflictions and "management" in such a way as to justify the exclusion of those personal, subjective issues in the patient, thereby immunizing medical personnel against the sense of vulnerability that inclusion of these issues might evoke. Thus, in addition to its bona fide scientific and therapeutic aspects—that is, its foundation in reality—biomedicine and other Western clinical specialties can be regarded as what Spiro (1965:100–113) called "culturally constituted defense mechanisms."

From a cultural viewpoint, the stories of sickness that correspond to the official, standardized formulas as to what constitutes a case seem, to their adherents, indeed complete. We shall argue in this volume that not only are such appearances deceptive, but that they are meant by their cultural actors to be precisely that, in order to ward off anxiety, aggressive impulses, guilt, shame, and threat to the coherence of the self. In exploring unconscious contributions to the story—both the underlying story and the defense system against recognizing it—we seek to further scientific knowledge and its application to clinical practice and teaching. We thus argue further that for stories of science to be scientific and not culture-bound, and for stories of healing to be genuinely therapeutic and not merely palliative or magically efficacious, they must be meta-cultural: that is, they must transcend the very cultures in which they are rooted.

A multitude of clinical stories are recited and played out in medical settings. Perhaps the most conspicuous is the sequence that consists of: the physician's accumulation of the patient's presenting complaint(s), medical/family/social/occupational histories (with the greatest attention being paid to the biomedical history and to the ostensibly genetic aspect of the family history); physical examination; laboratory and other high-technology tests; the formulation of a differential diagnosis (a list of the most probable diagnoses) and an eventual correct single diagnosis through the process of ruling out incorrect ones; the formulation of a treatment plan (clinical procedures, medication, etc.) that the physician prescribes for the patient; and finally, an outcome based on patient compliance with the regimen. Then there are more specialty-oriented stories: e.g., surgeons' preference for more invasive procedures; internists' and family physicians' preference for the prescribing of medication and other more conservative interventions; gastroenterologists' universe of the GI system; cardiologists' circumscribed world of the heart and circulatory system; pulmonologists' boundary around the lungs; and so forth. Hospital nurses end their story and responsibility toward the patient with the boundary of the hospital ("How can I get them well enough to go home?"); discharge planning and out patient follow-up ("What do they need when they go home?") are the domain, and tale, of other professions (home-health-care nurses, medical social workers, family-medicine clinic physicians, etc.). Home health care nurses' role expectations and patients' and families' expectations often differ markedly (Nurse: "There's only so much any one person can do, and you're spent"; Family: "You're here to take the pressure off us"; Patient: "I take my pills only when I feel sick").

Since the mid-1980s have been added Diagnosis Related Group (DRG)–based and Health Maintenance Organization (HMO)–based stories, "Doc-in-the-box" stories, and similar stories based on the bureaucratization or "McDonaldization" of medicine (Ritzer and Walczak 1986). The story of a hospitalized patient in the era of reimbursement based on diagnostic categories will be dictated in part by the maximum number of days the patient is permitted to be hospitalized according to the diagnosis. The limitation upon time is intrinsic to the physician's, the patient's, and the institution's story. As with all official stories or doctrines everywhere, there are with DRGs likewise folk variants: for instance, what is often called the DRG game, in which physicians, frustrated with hospital protocols and resulting limitations placed upon patient care, search among the various probable diagnoses for the one that would give the patient the longest allowable stay in the hospital.

Physicians (indeed, all health care personnel) and patients alike are influenced in their health care perceptions and decision making patterns by ethnic and religious beliefs. From the classic studies of Zborowski (1951, 1969), Barrabee and von Mering (1953), and Zola (1966) on various Euro-American ethnic groups, we learn that Irish Catholic patients are given to understatement if not denial of the severity of symptoms, whereas Italian Catholic patients tend to dramatize theirs; that the Irish tend to focus their symptoms on a single area of the body (e.g., eyes, ears, nose, or throat), while Italians tend to be more diffuse in their complaint of pain. European Jewish patients tend to search for deeper meanings and implications of symptoms and suffering, and tend not to be persuaded by an authoritative physician's pronouncements or reassurance; on the other hand, Italian-American patients are generally less concerned about the meaning of pains than with their immediate alleviation, as through analgesics. Although American physicians of various ethnicities perceive Jews and Italians both to be vociferous about their pains, they often fail to perceive that the purpose or function of the complaint differs between the groups.

Anglo-American (WASP) patients, like Jews, tend to be health-conscious, but attach very different significance to the search for health. Jews have been depicted as generally worried that something profoundly terrible might be wrong, whereas Anglo-Americans may be presented as viewing the body in a machinelike, utilitarian way: when something seems broken, one is obligated to take care of oneself and bring one's body to the doctor to be fixed. In this admittedly abbreviated ethnic construction of stories, Jews may see in the most minor symptom the harbinger of tragedy; Italians may primarily want to feel better and not bother thinking about taking the entire prescribed medical regimen; Irish patients might ignore their symptoms as long as possible, report only a few, and avoid the sense of sin that goes with too much preoccupation with the body; and WASP patients believe that rationality, hard work, control, and "pulling yourself up by your bootstraps" should work, in the treatment of disease as with the rest of life. Perhaps it is needless to say, but clinicians of all backgrounds bring and often unwittingly enact their ethnic-derived, reality-simplifying stories in patient care: i.e., how a good doctor and patient ought to act, what a good outcome ought to be, what degree of emotionality/ impersonality is appropriate, and so forth (Abel, Metraux, and Roll 1987). For example, many physicians drawn from and practicing among the farming/cowboy culture of the American Great Plains are intolerant of patients, especially males, who are more expressive than silently stoic and who take on the patient role for minor symptoms. In these physicians' stories, such patients are called wimps.

In traditional American biomedicine, the typical physician-patient relationship has been characterized by the patient offering a description of symptoms and their history, together with his or her body for examination and laboratory tests, to the physician who adduces the definitive "clinical picture"—the official story—from it. From this story, the physician recommends a course of action, with which the patient is expected to comply, thereby completing the physician's story as it "should" unfold. The patient's (and patient's family's and community's) own story is, in this official biomedical framework, incidental even if interesting. For the most part, patients' stories are viewed as signs of ignorance, bizarre or quaint thinking, or sheer mental illness—in any event, to be circumvented and not to be taken seriously except as obstacles to the completeness of the physician's own story.

In recent years, psychiatrist-anthropologist Arthur Kleinman, M.D., has proposed a clinical "negotiation" model (1978) to which he has given the name "explanatory models." According to this framework—one that has gained a modicum of acceptance in the biomedical literature—physician and patient alike (indeed all participants, from nurse to family) bring to the medical encounter both a general health-belief model (1980) and a situation-specific explanatory model. The latter consists of an etiological account, an explanation of the timing of onset of the symptoms, and an account of what is taking place and what should be done to remedy the situation. Kleinman labels the physician's model "disease" and the patient's model "illness."

Kleinman's model is part of a larger current within the disciplines of transcultural psychiatry and medical anthropology alike. Since the mid-1970s an influential ethnomedical school of thought has developed, of which such writers as Leon Eisenberg, Arthur Kleinman, Horacio Fabrega, Jr., Allan Young, Margaret Lock, and Nancy Scheper-Hughes are among the chief proponents. *Medical Anthropology Quarterly* and *Culture, Medicine, and Psychiatry* are two journals that give editorial emphasis to this hermeneutic approach that has for its focus "a truly social formulation of disease and its related phenomena" (Fabrega 1975: 969). Ethnomedical clinicians and writers study the "grammar" and "language" of clinical constructions (Fabrega 1975), as that of professional, folk, popular, and ethnic viewpoints alike. All participants to clinical encounters construct stories or narratives that are part of the construction of self in the negotiation of sickness roles.

It has been one of the major achievements of this ethnomedical school to argue widely and forcefully that biomedicine is itself an ethnomedical system, and its methods of data-collection and decision making constitute their own deeply cultural, not altogether culturally transcendent, story line. Fabrega, for instance, notes that "In Western cultures, 'disease' is what physicians and biologists study. The whole medical complex in Western nations, which includes knowledge, practices, organizations, and social roles, can be termed 'biomedicine.' Biomedicine thus constitutes our own culturally specific perspective about what disease is, and how medical treatment should be pursued; and like other medical systems, biomedicine is an interpretation which 'makes sense' in light of cultural traditions and assumptions about reality" (1975:969). He later adds that "Many of the problems in contemporary medical care that involve the relation of doctor to patient are outgrowths of the contrasting meanings that are given to disease by the participants" (ibid. 973). The clinical negotiation model propounded by Kleinman and colleagues represents an effort to arrive at a clinical consensus based on the joint construction of a common story line rather than the effort of the physician to impose a single story line.

Ideally, at least, the ethnomedical negotiation model differs markedly from the traditional biomedical story, in that the physician attempts to negotiate some common ground between the biomedical and the patient's stories rather than to impose the biomedical story while discounting that of the patient. According to Kleinman's view, in order to truly help the patient one must elicit, acknowledge (which is not the same as agreeing with), and attempt to work within the patient's own story. If we might transpose this into the work of pediatrician-psychoanalyst Donald W. Winnicott (1971), what occurs in the ideal Kleinman model is that physician and patient together create a new, common model within which they may work. Although the writers find much of value in the Kleinman model, we find that it is far too exclusively cognitive and secondary process-oriented. In order for physicians' and patients' explanatory models alike to be more complete, the Kleinman model needs to be both widened and deepened: that is, made more *dynamically interactive* so as to encompass the patient's and physician's social systems, and more *psychodynamically attuned* to incorporate the influence of all participants' mental structure on health perception and decision making. The great advance of the Kleinman model, however, must not be lost sight of in this criticism: that clinical work always consists of the interplay—the interpretation and misinterpretation—of the physician's and the patient's and others' stories.

The depth psychological approach taken throughout this volume deepens and supplements the cognitivist and constructivist social science schools, whose concepts such as presentation of self, cultural construction of illness, and health belief model are now widespread in the medical science literature. In our effort we urge the clinician of any specialty to shed the protective armor that knowing from the depths is dangerous. How else than shedding such armor can the clinician add strength to patients or families to help them confront otherwise painful and incompatible issues in their lives, issues that many an illness uncannily threatens to expose? Likewise, how else can any clinical teacher or supervisor urge a student or apprentice practitioner to grow beyond the lukewarm acceptable—and safe—notions of any period? This book builds on the authors' two prior volumes—*Context and Dynamics in Clinical Knowledge* (1985) and *From Metaphor to Meaning* (1987)—in our effort to render unconscious clinical stories more conscious, more accessible, and less toxic.

Consider the following two vignettes as examples of the complexity of clinical stories, and of the reasons that the breadth and depth of such stories are often opaque to narrator and listener (or interlocutor) alike.

VIGNETTE 1:
"MAYBE I'M IDENTIFYING WITH THE FATHER"

A family medicine intern, who also has a Ph.D. in clinical psychology and a notable work history in the state mental health department, presented to H. F. Stein the following case of a six-year-old girl dying of congenital enzymatic disorder.

> Her 6'4" father, wearing coveralls, and who states that he has three or four Ph.D.s, insists that he "knows" what's going on medically. He wants a "roundup" to kill all the bugs: "I want an X-ray," he tries to order. He constantly beeps the doctor, certain that there's something that can still be done to save his daughter. "I want her on everything, and now," he demands.
>
> The supervising physician is extremely irritated with the father, who threatens to call the hospital patient representative unless he gets his way. As intern, I'm only an observer in this case, but cases like this make me feel backed in the corner. At this point in our training we don't want

to admit "I don't know." The father calls the lab and knows the results before the nurses and doctors do. Rubs you wrong, demanding, wants everything done "my way." I want to refer these patients and fathers. You can feel their ANGER that something's wrong. She's going to die. What do you do with your own anger?

As an intern, you're lower than the patient. Losing control. The parent's intimidation and frustration plays on the doctor's frustration to gain control. What do you do, tell the patient to find another doctor? [Another intern added: "I'd rather have Dad be pushy than fall apart. I dread patients going boo-hoo. Sure we're taught to let them cry and grieve, but it makes you feel helpless just to stand there and do nothing. . . . What are we going to fill that void with when that boil bursts?"] So each intern puts in his time, and puts off talking with Dad about his grief: let the next intern take it. As soon as you start to get to know a patient or a family, your time's up. So you don't get involved, and just pass it on. It's easier on you that way.

[Another intern interjected: "What do you do if he CRIES? . . . Crying takes *time*. We're worried about residents and attendings seeing us just holding hands and comforting instead of acting like real doctors who are supposed to do something."] The parent wants control, the doctor wants control. The parent wants to take control from you. Interns have more problems with this, because they have absolutely no control in the hospital services. We don't even know if we can control *ourselves*.

Later on, privately, HFS as clinic consultant speculated to this same intern about yet another issue that might have upset him in this case—the fact that he himself had multiple higher education degrees, a notable professional work experience, and was now "just an intern," reduced to feeling like "a mole." His eyes brightened: "Maybe I'm really identifying with the father's sense of vulnerability and powerlessness. Maybe I see myself in his situation." Physician interns and residents, seasoned medical practitioners, indeed, clinicians of all types, are especially emotionally vulnerable to overidentification with and revulsion toward patients whose life situations and stages are similar to theirs and who evoke in them what they are struggling to repress. Here, the angry and frightened father of the patient was feeling helpless and being demanding—feelings and actions that the intern, seeking to be professional and well-controlled, could neither acknowledge nor show. HFS learned later that this intern's wife was at that time pregnant with their first child, a fact that might have added to the identification. The intern's outrage at this parent's obnoxiousness almost literally melted from his face as he came to realize and feel more fully himself how helpless, humiliated, and enraged *he* felt as a "mere" intern—just as the patient's perhaps multiply-degreed father had felt himself to be a "mere" father, powerless to save his daughter.

Let us offer a second vignette, this time from surgery. It might be thought that unconscious, family-of-origin issues in physicians might affect and interfere with their ability to deal with patients' psychosocial or psychiatric difficulties (as in vignette 1, central themes of which were helplessness, death and dying, vulnerability), but certainly they do not taint the more seemingly "hard," "objective," processes of biomedical diagnosis and treatment. In a recent paper, Smith and Stein (1987) have argued that out-of-awareness physician factors can distort *any* clinical process.

VIGNETTE 2:
THE SURGEON'S CERTAINTY

In a poignant vignette, physician-psychoanalyst Jay Katz illustrates how unconscious Oedipal factors in a surgeon, George Crile, Jr., affected his eager embracing of radical mastectomy as a means of totally denying uncertainty.

Crile [Jr.] wrote that his father, George Crile, Sr., a renowned surgeon of the early twentieth century under whom he trained, *"never* did a radical mastectomy" [Crile 1973]. Instead, his father always employed a less mutilating surgical procedure. George Crile, Jr., continued, "during my residency at the Cleveland Clinic, I was also exposed to the influence of Dr. Tom Jones, who *always* did a radical mastectomy. Being a rebellious child, I discounted my father's ideas, adopted the Jones technique, and for seventeen years I performed only radical mastectomies." Now, however, Crile concluded, "conventional radical mastectomies are not done" at the Cleveland Clinic.

Having been trained by his father and Jones, Crile was aware of the uncertainties that surrounded the proper treatment of breast cancer, but he was compelled to deny uncertainty and substitute an uncompromising certainty in its place for powerful personal reasons. His conversion raises many questions. In now following his father, has he merely become a compliant child? How can he know? Or, put differently, to what extent can he demand that patients trust him implicitly since he was so readily affected by oedipal conflicts, which he fought out over the bodies of countless Jocastas? Indeed, to what extent do many surgeons, trained by other illustrious "fathers," replicate this struggle by performing only procedures prescribed by their elders' paternal authority, to which they submit passively because they have not sufficiently resolved their conflicts with their biological fathers? I enlist these psychological considerations both to emphasize how these and other powerful forces can defeat an awareness of uncertainty and to encourage a more self-conscious and reflective recognition of the constant presence of uncertainty in medical practice. Such heightened awareness may alert physicians to the fact that something may be amiss whenever single-mindedness dominates their therapeutic interventions. (Katz 1984:38)

It will be our thesis throughout this book that storytelling and listening between clinician and patient (or client, family, fellow clinician, and staff member) can *facilitate or prohibit the emergence of the deeper intrapsychic story.* Ironically and sadly, one of the latent functions of clinical practice is often to protect the clinician from the painful reemergence of his or her own intrapsychic story via the patient. Patient care often serves as an interpersonal defense mechanism. Thus, often precisely what the patient needs to be healed if not cured (in the biomedical sense) is precisely what the clinician defends against in himself or herself most. In *Countertransference and Psychotherapeutic Technique,* for example, James Masterson admonishes therapists that "To the degree to which you have not resolved your own depression (not necessarily an abandonment depression), you will have great difficulty tolerating your patient's depression, because it stimulates your own. It resonates with a lot of the things which you experienced as a child which you have repressed, and it stimulates them and starts tugging on them; they start pushing up, trying to get release" (1983:188). For clinician (therapist, physician, etc.) and patient alike, the implicit and explicit stories *together* constitute the "whole" story (technically: the defenses or resistance, the transference and countertransference, and the underlying affects, fantasies, and reconstructed traumata). Moreover, the mental organization of clinician and patient alike will determine the "choice" of story (similar to symptom choice) that can be articulated, elicited, or heard. It will be a theme throughout this book that only as the clinician can tolerate to experience his or her underlying story, can he or she tolerate and foster the unfolding of the patient's story—and hence foster the greater integration of both rather than defend against the return of the split-off and repressed by finding ways to get rid of the patient or to limit treatment to validating or proving those stories that reinforce the defenses.

Family physician and philosopher Howard Brody recently writes that "we cannot understand a right and good healing action without understanding what the sickness is doing to the person's self-respect, to his life plan, and to the narrative account of his life. One characteristic of a story is that it clearly makes sense and hangs together once it has been told" (Brody 1987: 192). The chapters in this volume are about the subtleties and nuances of patients' and families' stories and their interplay with both the resistance and the accessibility practitioners of all clinical vocations have to these stories. In the chapters to follow, the psychoanalytic-ethnographic approach to patient care, clinical teaching, and clinical supervision will be described and illustrated in much detail. It provides the foundation on which securing the story behind the story is built.

ORGANIZATION OF THIS VOLUME

This volume is divided into two sections: I: Clinical Work: Patients, Families, and Their Stories, and II: Stories and Their Translations in Clinical Education and Supervision.

In a sense the emphasis in the first section is the most traditional and conventional: that of empathy and persistence with individual patients, their families, and other key figures in their personal network to uncover the stories underlying and sustaining the pathology. Stated another way, we explore symptoms and their significance in the customary categories known as "patients" or "clients," people who present themselves as having (or being) problems, people who are diagnosed by clinicians (and often by their families and occupational or community networks as well), and whom health and mental health professionals treat.

In the second section, we turn our attention to the stories that practitioners—as individuals, as members of work groups, and as members of clinical institutions—bring to clinical encounters and construct during patient care or therapy. These stories, from the idiosyncratic to the officially taught, often interfere with the clinician's ability to hear and to elicit the patient's (or family's) story. In this second section, we offer a psychoanalytically informed ethnographic training model for helping clinicians of all disciplines to gain greater access to their own inner stories and thereby to distort less the patient's and family's story.

REFERENCES

Abel, T. M., R. Metraux, and S. Roll. 1987. *Psychotherapy and culture,* revised and expanded edition. Albuquerque: University of New Mexico Press.

Barrabee, P., and O. von Mering. 1953. Ethnic variations in mental stress in families with psychotic children. *Social Problems* 1:48–53.

Boyer, L. B. 1979. *Childhood and folklore: A psychoanalytic study of Apache personality.* New York: The Library of Psychological Anthropology.

Brody, H. 1987. *Stories of sickness.* New Haven, Conn.: Yale University Press.

Crile, G., Jr. 1973. How much surgery for breast cancer? *Modern Medicine* 41 (12):32–38.

Fabrega, H., Jr. 1975. The need for an ethnomedical science. *Science* 189 :969–75.

Ferreira, A. J. 1963. Family myth and homeostasis. *Archives of General Psychiatry* 9:55–61.

Grolnick, S. 1987. Reflections on psychoanalytic subjectivity and objectivity as applied to anthropology. *Ethos* 15(1):136–43.

Katz, J. 1984. Why doctors don't disclose uncertainty. *The Hastings Center Report* 14(1):35–44.

Kleinman, A. 1978. Relevance of anthropological and cross-cultural research: Concepts and strategies. *American Journal of Psychiatry* 135:427–31.

——. 1980. *Patients and healers in the context of culture: An exploration of the borderland between anthropology, medicine, and psychiatry.* Berkeley and Los Angeles: University of California Press.

Kris, E. 1956. The personal myth—A problem in psychoanalytic technique. *Journal of American Psychoanalytic Association* 4:653–81.

Masterson, J. F. 1983. *Countertransference and psychotherapeutic technique: Teaching seminars on psychotherapy of the borderline adult.* New York: Brunner/Mazel.

Munson, R. 1981. Why medicine cannot be a science. *Journal of Medicine and Philosophy* 6:183–208.

Ritzer, G., and D. Walczak. 1986. The changing nature of American medicine. *Journal of American Culture* 9(4):43–51.

Smith, R. C., and H. F. Stein. 1987. A topographical model of clinical decision making and interviewing. *Family Medicine* 19(5):361–63.

Spiro, M. E. 1965. Religious systems as culturally constituted defense mechanisms. In *Context and meaning in cultural anthropology,* edited by M. E. Spiro, 100–113. New York: The Free Press.

——. 1982. Preface to the second edition of his *Buddhism and society: A great tradition and its Burmese vicissitudes,* xi–xix. Berkeley and Los Angeles: University of California Press (orig. 1970).

Stein, H. F., and M. Apprey. 1985. *Context and dynamics in clinical knowledge,* vol. 1 of the Series in Ethnicity, Medicine, and Psychoanalysis. Charlottesville: University Press of Virginia.

——. 1987. *From metaphor to meaning: Papers in psychoanalytic anthropology,* vol. 2 of the Series in Ethnicity, Medicine, and Psychoanalysis. Charlottesville: University Press of Virginia.

Stierlin, H. 1973. Group fantasies and family myths: Some theoretical and practical aspects. *Family Process* 12:111–25.

Whitehead, A. N. 1960. *Religion in the making.* Cleveland and New York: Meridian (orig. 1926).

Winnicott, D. W. 1971. *Playing and reality.* New York: Basic Books.

Zborowski, M. 1951. Cultural components in responses to pain. *Journal of Social Issues* 8:16–30.

——. 1969. *People in pain.* San Francisco: Jossey-Bass.

Zola, I. K. 1966. Culture and symptoms: An analysis of patient's presenting complaints. *American Sociological Review* 31:615–30.

PART I

Clinical Work:
Patients, Families, and
Their Stories

CHAPTER 1

What Is Therapeutic In Clinical Relationships?

HOWARD F. STEIN

DOCTOR AS THERAPIST

The subject of this chapter is that nebulous realm of clinical interaction and outcome that currently goes by the scientifically doleful name of nonspecific, the sine qua non of therapeutic effect. From some fifteen years' work with psychiatry and family medicine residents, I have frequently been the object of an anxious and angry outcry: "Too much analysis is just paralysis. Don't just help me to understand the case. Tell me what to do, so that I can get in there, intervene, make things better quickly, and finish. All you leave me is impotence. Where does this leave me? This sort of analysis just makes things worse. I would rather *not* know so much. You end up not being able to do anything."

Many residents have protested to me and to other behavioral science colleagues over the years: "I went to medical school and into residency training to become a doctor, to cure disease, not to become a therapist or counselor." The very terms *therapist* and *counselor* often feel inimical to the self-perception and identity of a physician—not only in what one does in the role but in what sort of person one is in that role. For many, the appurtenances of the medical profession are used as a form of protection against being too disturbed or touched by the patient (or rather, by what the patient represents in oneself and one's past). In a phrase, for many doctoring is a role-implemented defense against the dangers of being in a therapeutic relationship.

One young family physician, having successfully gotten his patient into and through surgery, said as much from sheer relief as from pride: "Finally I found a real disease I could do something about. . . . The more you get into areas you can't do anything about, the more frustrated you get." Values of mastery, doing, curing, winning, simplifying, and conquering are all part of the physician role that students and residents have in mind (Kluckhohn and Strodtbeck 1961). Conversely, they regard values associated with the therapist and the counselor role as more interpersonal and reflective; more involved with being and becoming than sheer, aggressive doing; as emphasizing listening, empathy, comforting, "communication" rather than "action"; and as involving a more intimate knowledge of and association with the patient and the family than the instrumental role of the physician requires. Therefore, they find these values to be only of limited use, overemphasized, uncomfortable, and occasionally repugnant. They do not want to stand back, look, feel, analyze, and wait; rather they wish to "get in there and stamp out disease."

Although, in our culture, physicians seem to draw a distinction between the practice of "real medicine" and that of "therapy" or "counseling" (while other helping professionals vigorously distinguish further between therapy and counseling!), the deeper contrast should be between what is therapeutic and what is antitherapeutic in any form of communication. The question is—for any relationship: "Is the relationship itself therapeutic or antitherapeutic?" Thus, the presence of therapy lies, not in the name or degree of the clinician's role and qualifications, but in the character of the relationship itself: that is, whether we stretch ourselves toward another or we withdraw from others and hide behind theory, procedure, or technique of *any* sort. To be clinically therapeutic with a patient, for instance, one must find the patient to be interesting—in his or her own right, not merely the container of an interesting disease or an intrusion to be gotten rid of as soon as possible. Measures to reduce the amount of time and personal involvement with a patient have taken root throughout modern medicine. Yet it is personal commitment that is the bedrock of all that is ultimately therapeutic—"For thou art with me," says the psalmist in his darkest moment.

One is either therapeutic or antitherapeutic in any kind of relationship or situation. And learning to hone the distinction takes at least a lifetime. We either heal or we injure, nurture integration or sow the seeds of fragmentation, foster maturity or regression, treat the other truly as another (that is, as a subject) or treat the other as some extension of ourselves (that is, as an object and receptacle). We can allow ourselves a growing sense of intimacy with our own inner recesses and thereby increase the ease of our intimacy with patients, family, colleagues, residents, and students; or we can use the teaching and practice of medicine as a defense against ourselves and others.

SELF AND SUBJECT IN MEDICINE

Since *what we do* is inseparable from *who we are* and *what we mean*—either unconsciously or consciously—it behooves us when considering the clinical relationship to incorporate an interest in the physician's own identity and meanings. Whether our intervention—of any kind—will be therapeutic or antitherapeutic depends upon what we do with our anxiety. We can use our intervention to flee into action in order not to know and feel, or we first can use our very anxiety to know and feel. Then we can include this additional knowledge as part of our plan of action. To be therapeutic, we simply must have access to data about ourselves that will permit us to have access to similar data in patients, residents, staff members, and students. This does not supplant biomedical knowledge and skills; rather, it supplements it with a different level and type of knowledge. Without the latter, one may inadvertently misuse official knowledge and skills in what Langs (1978) calls a "therapeutic misalliance."

We Americans have an ongoing love affair with efficiency, brevity, streamlining, paring things down to size. These attitudes and sometimes virtues have taken us far. But, with people as with nature, they can also get us in trouble. In medicine such attitudes unwittingly lead us to diminish and dishonor patients, families, doctors, and staff alike. Medicine risks becoming something of an unfeeling plant assembly line, the primary goal of which is to "move 'em up and move 'em out." In our brave new world of Diagnostic Related Groups (DRGs) and Peer Review Organizations (PROs), I suppose that the resulting clinical shortcut could be "evaluated" to be effective. But it should not be confused with anything therapeutic, since the care of the patient no longer occupies the highest priority. Therapy, on the other hand, takes time, money, and commitment. Disingenuously, shortcuts rationalized according to the logic of briefer and briefer therapies only short-circuit therapy by disavowing maturity as a worthy goal and compassion as a worthy attitude.

I have heard countless physicians say, both in fact and in essence: "I should be able to change the patient; I have an obligation to change the patient; the patient should be willing to change, otherwise, Why does the patient come to the doctor? And if I can't change the patient, I'm a failure." We are preparing our young doctors for an unrealistic attitude toward themselves and their patients, and the failure of realism is antitherapeutic. To expect and train a physician to be infallible, totally responsible, omniscient, omnipotent, omnibenevolent, absolutely certain, and always decisive is dangerous to the health of doctor, patient, and society alike— even if society demands perfection from its physicians. To be in a therapeutic position, the physician can empathetically acknowledge the wishes and expressed needs of his or her patient, but must at times frustrate and fail to satisfy many of them in the service of the greater maturity of all participants (Gutheil, Bursztajn, and Brodsky 1984). The effort to be patient pleasers on the one hand, and to exact compliance from patients on the other hand, are twin countertherapeutic seductions of modern medicine.

In his essay on "Dialogue," Martin Buber wrote that:

> Genuine responsibility exists only where there is real responding.
> Responding to what?
> To what happens to one, to what is to be seen and heard and felt.
> Each concrete hour allotted to the person, with its content drawn from the world and from destiny, is speech for the man who is attentive. (1965:16)

In *I and Thou* he wrote that "Magic desires to obtain its effects without entering into relation, and practises its tricks in the void" (1958:83). The relationship between doctor and patient always stands at risk of subversion by the patient's wish to receive and by the physician's desire to produce, a magical prescription that dissolves relation into substance or technique alone. Now, what separates scientific prescription from magical prescription is, not the pharmacological content, but the implied intention of the act. When antibiotic or advice is administered or presented as a magic bullet, doctor or patient or both have forsaken the realm of science for magic, the presence of I and Thou for the manipulations of one It to another. The patient compliance or patient satisfaction thus achieved are fleeting bursts of infantile omniscience, omnipotence, (received or bestowed) omnibenevolence and infallibility. Such magic "exists" only in the earliest mental world where gesture commands the world that is its extension. In this world there are only deeds, not people. The physician can understand this regressive pull both in himself or herself and in the patient—but to indulge it is to forsake people for things. Medicine that heals—not that tricks—is always contained within the clinical relationship (Balint 1957). The relationship itself is the act of healing: the healer, who has learned to forego magic, helps the patient to become healed or reconciled to life's irreversibility and loss's irrevocability by first declining to comply with the patient's request for magic. The physician's prescription and his/her presence need not be antithetical, so long as they serve reality while fully acknowledging wish. The more physicians can trust their disclosure of presence, the less they will feel called upon—by themselves or by patients—to outwit patients rather than to address them. Clinicians must be constantly prepared for unexpected symbolic turns of meanings, for patients or families will be able to endure, feel, and understand their own anxiety and defenses only to the extent that they believe the clinician feels safe enough with this unsettling material. The physician must thus be willing to *accompany* and *let go of* the patient, as much as to *lead* and *direct* the patient when the occasion calls for it.

TECHNIQUE AND DEFENSE

In medicine, our watchwords include being "in control" if not "in charge." Yet a decade and a half in graduate medical education—much of which has been spent on the front lines (to borrow from medicine's military metaphor) with psychiatry and family medicine residents, their patients, families, and staffs—has taught me also the courage of chaos, of ambiguity, of uncertainty, of waiting. Each time I listen to a resident or see a patient and resident (or family) together, I bring with me everything I believe I know, and attempt to listen afresh as if I know nothing. For the truth of the matter is that we never know beforehand what it is that we need to know, or look for or hear, let alone do. If a resident is to have the courage of chaos—for the sake of the patient—and trust that order will ultimately emerge—then I too as educator must learn this same dauntlessness for the sake of the resident (and secondarily the patient or family). It is as if medicine is created anew with each patient encounter and physician consultation. It is not enough, I have come to teach, to merely "practice" medicine—if by *practice* we mean the application of what we know as the state of the art. Technique must be responsive to our capacity to learn something new from reality—which includes the patient, our best teacher. Simplified diagnoses and automatically applied techniques are our signs and symptoms of defense against what we fear to know—about ourselves in the guise of the patient.

I have no quarrel with technique per se (from surgery to medication to confrontation to paradox). Yet even here technique is inseparable from the conscious and unconscious uses for which it is invented in the first place and later applied. At issue in clinical and research matters alike is "the *unconscious use* of sound methodological devices *primarily* as defense mechanisms and only *incidentally* as (sublimatory) scientific techniques" (Devereux 1967:100). The trouble is that we can design scientific techniques for dereistic purposes that protect us from the very data we need in order to comprehend and act. The authentic healer, I have learned, is not the one with the answers before the questions are posed, but the one who can bear the anxiety of pursuing questions rather than rushing to answers. This healer is not the Aristotelean unmoved mover, but the most moved mover. One who can heal is one who can first allow oneself to be moved, touched—nay, wounded—by the patient. In fact as in etymology, to be a patient is to suffer. To heal is first to acknowledge that suffering.

THE WOUNDED HEALER

In the Blanchard Lecture, G. Gayle Stephens, M.D., argued that: "Pellegrino [Pellegrino and Thomasma 1982] has written that the fundamental characteristic of clinical medicine is wounded humanity seeking cure at the hands of a physician. This is not the same as a consumer purchasing a commodity. The therapeutic relationship has never been equal. Woundedness makes the difference. The contract is not enough, there must be a covenant that goes beyond what anyone has a right to demand and that cannot be compensated with money" (1984: 15). Now, the allegory of "wounded humanity" has as its parallel the image of the archetypal physician Asklepios as the wounded healer, that is, one who is capable of being profoundly moved by the patient's suffering and is thereby able to address its depth (Kerenyi 1959).

During the past decade, the consumerist or patients' rights movement, on the one hand, and the industrialization or corporatization of the medical profession, on the other, can at least in part be understood to be a retreat on the part of patients, practitioners, and public alike from the vulnerabilities of wounded humanity. They approach medical care as though it were a commodity to be traded for, the human body a machine, the human mind a computer, and the clinical relationship an impersonal exchange of computerized information. Dissatisfaction with an emotionally if not functionally hierarchical relationship had led not only to an emphasis on individualism and a demand for a more equal "partnership" in the clinical relationship but to an adversarial competition for one-upmanship in the guise of equality.

Perhaps needless to say, the exercise of authoritarianism in the guise of individualism (Spiegel 1971), and the resort to what Bateson (1972) called "symmetrical" escalations in one's approach to problem solving, are hardly limited to medicine and its constituency, but, in fact, are American cultural patterns. The history of management and labor, and of various ethnic groups vying for equality (Stein and Hill 1977), reads much like the recent history of medicine in the U.S.A., each component feeling a sense of entitlement for various grievances, each wishing for vengeance for having been wronged, and each going on the defensive and the offensive to protect what it sees as its endangered interests. There can be no common ground when both sides of the ideological tracks come to see each other as personifying evil. Each *protects* rather than *exposes* his/her own wounded humanity.

Life is deep, and so, therefore, must medicine be. Work in family medicine and psychiatry departments has brought me daily face-to-face with my own subjectivity, and how everything I do and say bears the footprint of my biography. Rather than recoil from that fact, I try to gain increasing access to it and to use it. I attempt to reach outward toward a resident or patient by being able to reach inward without fearing loss of reality or of my self. I have had to learn to trust that which my childhood, family, and education had trained me to forget. I have learned that the more I permit myself to reclaim of my past, the more I can permit patients or students to "have" of their past.

As medical educators or physicians, we are always making disclosures about ourselves. The pictures and knickknacks in our offices, the choices of office decor and waiting-room furniture, the selection of magazines and handouts in the reception area, the colleagues with whom we consult and to whom we refer patients and families—these are profound, value-laden, personal disclosures. What is more, quite apart from what words or stories their doctors bestow, patients are constantly "borrowing" as well: defenses, insights, and wisdom alike. The question is, What is the physician making available to the patient, both consciously and unconsciously?

The self of the physician—of any clinician—is a powerful diagnostic and therapeutic tool. In permitting intimacy and reciprocity through the use of the self in medicine, the clinician is acknowledging a shared, common humanity with the patient, despite the necessity of divided function and unequal roles (Candib 1987). In offering oneself and one's own experiences and feelings, the clinician is serving as a provider of a feeling or of affect-ridden memory that is currently missing or out of awareness in the patient. In offering oneself, the clinician helps the patient to remember and thereby to become more whole. The reverse is likewise true, as Searles wrote in "The Patient as Therapist to His Analyst" (1975). To heal is not only to ply a trade or a technique. It is to be moved by the one whom one would heal. Attentive listening is itself an act of intimacy and reciprocity. One tells or discloses much about oneself by what one can and cannot afford to allow the patient to say or to permit oneself to hear and respond to.

We talk sloppily and glibly about maintaining a "therapeutic position," of meting out "acceptance" and "reframing" and "paradox," as if posture were equivalent to stature, as if a false mask could ever pass for a true face. But only one who can truly take a stand can help another stand as well. And the ability to meet a patient face-to-face rests upon the ability to face oneself—in the mirror of one's memory and as the patient mirrors oneself as well. One can truly recognize a patient only if one is willing to recognize oneself in the patient (to use projective identification in an empathetic, rather than a rejecting, way). It is not enough to acquire clinical skills and techniques, for know-how does not exist apart from *what it is used for*—and that brings us back to the clinician and the relationship once again (Smith and Stein 1987). This is not therapeutic solipsism or narcissism: it is life.

The physician's power does not reside in the command of technique alone but in the ability to comprehend the depths of the patient's life, which enables the physician to understand in turn the significance of the illness to the patient. Any formulation of "comprehensive care" that omits the dimension of *comprehending* the patient omits the whole of the patient's life and reduces it to fragmentariness—even if the heap of fragments is deceptively immense. It is not only that we have so much to do to patients; but that we have so much to learn from them—that, in turn, alters the face of assessment, diagnosis, treatment, and outcome. And I can only claim this from having learned to bear witness to it in myself. I *learned to teach* by learning to listen to residents rather than rushing to be their "provider" with answers or formulas. For, paradoxically, "answers" can be part of the problem and often prevent us from peering more deeply and broadly into the abyss. Increasingly, I have come to teach residents—and through them, perhaps, patients—what the residents have unwittingly just taught me. The inventor of the stethoscope, Lannec, is reputed to have admonished his students: "Listen to your patient, he is telling you what is wrong with him."

Patients may grievously err in their interpretation of their symptoms, but if we follow their symbolic pathways as diligently as we do neurological ones, they cannot but lead us to where we both may have feared to go. The rabbit hole into Wonderland is the royal road to healing.

A therapeutic environment, then, is not one that stereotypically relies upon "doing" in our cultural sense of aggressive intervention, but rather is one that is also capable of integrating within the clinical repertory the ability to accompany and follow the patient's lead into the wonderland of the patient's own life situation and meanings. One resident recently wisely said that "One of the hardest things to know is when to do nothing." Of course, here, *doing* gains its meaning from a larger frame of reference. In avoiding the trap imposed by oneself, one's family of origin, one's medical education, and one's patients to "do something" simply because one is the doctor, one can instead withstand and absorb the patient's anxiety rather than act in order to rid oneself of it. Attentive to the patient's needs, the provider provides a safe, protective "holding environment" (Modell 1976) in which the patient feels understood. Whatever else one may elect to do clinically, the "listening process" (Langs 1978) and its attendant "regression in the service of the other" (Olinick 1969) remain the foundation of the entire clinical edifice. And while these certainly involve self-discipline and the learning of interviewing and diagnostic skills, they rest ultimately upon the clinician's interest in the patient, attentiveness to the patient, compassion for the patient, commitment to the patient, and finally the clinician's fine-honed ability to tolerate, understand, and utilize his/her emotional arousal by the patient (Volkan 1981).

To help establish the distinction between therapeutic and countertherapeutic uses of self in medicine, it is also instructive to recall Freud's own reasons for insisting on the analyst's neutrality and abstinence (1914:164–66). Freud had already developed the techniques of uncovering the unconscious complexes and analyzing patients' resistance to such insight—only to have many of his female patients begin professing their love for him. He concluded that the analyst "must recognize that the patient's falling in love is induced by the analytic situation and is not to be attributed to the charms of his own person . . ." (1914:160–61). Whereupon Freud placed the analysis of the patient's transference at the core of psychoanalysis.

What Freud courageously concludes revolutionized not only technique but the very understanding of what the patient needs. Because the goal of the therapeutic relationship is to help the patient master his or her own life, "it is quite out of the question for the analyst to give way. However highly he may prize love he must prize even more highly the opportunity for helping his patient over a decisive stage in her life" (1910:170). Now, falling in love with one's patient is but one of countless temptations in clinical work. The crucial ethical, technical, and relational question is whether a specific use of the clinician's self constitutes his or her *own* resistance to the patient's therapy, mastery, and hence greater autonomy, or whether it fosters it.

Intimacy and reciprocity are hardly limited to whether the clinician discloses some anecdote about himself or herself, or about his or her own life. Disclosure, or defense against it, is revealed in the clinician's very attentiveness and responsiveness to the patient and/or the family. The empathetic use of the self in clinical work, or its opposite, the selective withholding or withdrawal of empathy from the patient by becoming obsessed with medical procedure or by punitively "firing" the patient, already constitutes an act of self-disclosure that allows or forbids the patient's own self-revelation to the doctor. That having been said, I must add at once that it is often unbearably difficult to listen receptively to patients and to hear their suffering (which is not the same as "fixing" their disease). Patients themselves may well conceal their suffering for their own self-protective reasons. Once heard, it is difficult to respond to patient's suffering with the insight of our common vulnerability rather than with fight or flight.

In addition to there being powerful individual and professionally inculcated (consolidated into a professional superego, as it were) forces that militate against intimacy and reciprocity in clinical relationships, there have been added in recent years malignant institutional and cultural ones as well. A societywide attitude of social Darwinism, militarism, nationalism, nuclear provocation, survivalism, withdrawal of compassion and responsibility—of which obsession with economic "bottom lines" is but a symptom and metaphor—contributes an especially alluring group permissiveness to what is already a personal and professional proclivity. In the current social climate of regressively frenzied self-seeking, I have heard many contend, Who ever said we owed them (patients, the poor, the middle-class, the planet?) anything?

Intimacy and reciprocity require a willingness to expose one's own vulnerability to another. Yet the political-economic-cultural mood encourages, if anything, the exploitation of others' vulnerability in the service of protecting oneself. Intimacy and reciprocity presuppose time and commitment, qualities that seem inimical to corporate—not to say national—priorities. In this conflict we, as medical professionals and laypersons alike, must now choose between being healers and being destroyers. The doctor-patient relationship is but one forum in which that momentous choice is being made.

CULTURAL ISSUES AND
THE NATURE OF THERAPY

In this final section, I address the thorny issues of the relationship between culture and healing, for I take the nonrelativistic position that all that goes by the name healing in whatever social group is not necessarily therapeutic—for identified patient, clinician, or the group itself.

In a courageous paper, "Approaching Cross-Cultural Psychotherapy," Boyer discusses the "discrepancy between the patient's and the therapist's therapeutic goals" (1983:237) based upon his thirty-five years of practice as a psychoanalyst in the San Francisco area and twenty-five years of research among the Apaches. Communication style and culturally patterned expectations often differ between patient and therapist. Boyer identifies elements in Apache shamanistic philosophy that are widely shared in faith-healing beliefs and practices of all groups: e.g., the interlacing of religion, medical practices, mythology, and folklore; the capacity of the shaman to use his supernatural power for good (healing) or for bad (witchcraft to bring harm to others); the use of laying on of hands, administration of herbs, prestidigitation, etc., which "serve essentially to enhance the patient's belief in the curer's omnipotence. In many cultures hallucinogens and consciousness altering drugs are used for that purpose and to reduce the patient's capacity to think logically" (1983:239).

From a cross-cultural point of view, La Barre (1975) writes that a shaman's treatment of disease caused by "possession" by an alien spirit is exorcism. "The Navajo night chanter uses a ground painting in which to cast the disease spirit, and afterward the painting is destroyed" (1975:15). Once the painting is erased, the malevolent cause of disease is magically dispelled and dispersed. While the conscious representation of the repressed is temporarily effaced, the unconscious conflict remains, requiring subsequent visits to the putative curer. True, such curing rites reintegrate the individual into society; but since the devils that have been cast out remain latently and valently within (where they have always been a split-off

part of the self), they are prepotent causes of further stress, neces-
sitating subsequent treatment and the permanence of the curing
role. Likewise, despite the financially costly and often physically
painful process of reassurance, the patient who began by the conversion of anxiety into imagined or real somatic pain retains the
source of anxiety that has gone unattended by a ritual aimed at
avoiding the shared unconscious source of the conflict. Ritual cure
can therefore never resolve conflict, since it is dependent on the
persistence of the conflict it aims to remove.

A number of psychoanalytic researchers have noted how therapies tend to be culturally fixed in the vicious circle of pathology and
symptom remission. On the basis of Opler's (1936) work among the
Apache, Devereux (1980) comments that "Apache shamans can
cure tics (which are notoriously resistant to psychotherapy) by sub-
stituting a taboo for the tic. . . . What seems to happen in such
'cures' is simply a changeover from idiosyncratic conflicts and defenses to culturally conventional conflicts and ritualized symptoms,
without any real curative insight" (1980: 17–18).

Boyer (1983) compares and contrasts faith healing and insight-
oriented psychotherapy. He argues that while in faith healing, diagnosis is irrelevant and reliance upon supernatural force essential, in
Western psychiatry diagnosis is essential. The insight-oriented therapist relies on evidence that emerges from the data and from the
therapeutic alliance rather than from belief that in turn is used to
confirm preexisting belief. "He sees the patient's wish to view him as
omnipotent as part of transference phenomena and his aim is to
free the patient both of transference distortions and of his relationship with the therapist. He knows that abrupt symptom removal
frequently disguises underlying psychopathology. He views suggestion therapy to be not infrequently a manifestation of countertransference problems" (1983:239–40).

Boyer urges that the therapist be interested in and cognizant of
"the style, content and implications of [the patient's] verbal and
nonverbal communications" (1983:240), and be especially attentive
to culturally based discrepancies between the therapist's and client's
expectations, for often the "patient hopes for cure through faith
healing" (1983:240). Successful therapy "requires mutual understanding of verbal and nonverbal messages by the therapist and the
patient" (1983:241).

The significance of Boyer's paper for family practitioners and
other physicians lies in the continuity of certain aspects of faith
healing *within* the biomedical tradition, not merely historically pre-

ceding or outside it. One can think of many powerful vestiges of the magical in modern scientific guise: the routine B-12 and penicillin shots given to patients upon demand; the aura of the sacred that patients and physicians alike confer upon the high technology of medicine; the expectation of instant cure by the "magic bullet" that must be ritually prescribed at the conclusion of the office visit; the medical equation of symptom removal with cure; frequent reliance upon suggestion, optimism, and reassurance to mobilize a patient's hope, and to generate patient compliance and satisfaction; the significance to patient, family, and medical staff alike of medical symbolism that heightens clinical authority.

Boyer's paper serves as a timely reminder of how in all medicine the wish to heal and the wish to he healed interact. While physicians in the biomedical tradition are not merely contemporary shamans, the many parallels in expectation and function are too great to discount. Boyer's brief but synoptic article contributes to our understanding of the psychodynamics of any clinical relationship, and therefore to the current debate over what is precisely *therapeutic*.

My only caveat with Boyer is with his view of diagnosis, for intrinsic to all healing endeavors is the identification or labeling and explanation of the malady (Kleinman 1980). Action always follows naming. In faith healing, diagnosis is never entirely absent and irrelevant; rather, diagnosis is not allowed to penetrate the symbolic veneer to the core of the pain. Diagnosis colludes with patient, family, and community *not* to penetrate it, but only to manipulate and resymbolize it in ways that reaffirm everyone's defenses.

In critically evaluating any clinical decision-making process—the biomedical included—one must inquire into what types of data serve as evidence and what types are excluded, and why. In faith healing, the symbolic reality and authority of the healer *must* be upheld. In psychodynamically oriented healing, which ideally also includes the physician, the symbolic reality of both healer and client are constantly explored for their latent meanings. With benevolent skepticism, the insightful physician asks himself/herself what the faith healer cannot tolerate asking: What is diagnosis for? Whom does the diagnosis (and treatment) serve? Diagnostic belief on the part of patient and family and clinician alike can easily be a rationalized form of resistance to self-knowledge, which obscures the pathological process occurring in the patient under the guise of illuminating it. What Boyer so lucidly describes as a contrast between two *types of healers* characterizes, I believe, an inner polarity *within* modern scientific medicine itself.

On the basis of the ethnographic record, it has become a truism in anthropology that the "medical" component or system of a culture is enmeshed in the ethos of that culture, which pervades all institutions. For instance, writing of "Morita Therapy" in Japan, Kiefer observes that: "Morita Therapy is . . . a kind of cultural institution, subject to the same influences that shape other institutions in this society. . . . Even the types of neurotic disorder for which the technique is most often used . . . are the sort which one would expect to flourish in the Japanese social atmosphere. In short, the study of a treatment modality tells us a surprising amount about the society in which it is practiced" (1976:11).

The structure of relationships in healing settings parallels the preferred structure of relationships in other social institutions as well (e.g., family, religious, political). Thus, Draguns (1981) argues that cultures with authoritarian political systems tend not to have much individual psychotherapy as preferred modes of treatment. And Wintrob (1973) argues that societies with strong authority structure tend to use magic to explain and treat mental disorders. What can be said to characterize supposedly whole cultures can also be said for different historical eras in the same culture. In our own time in the U.S.A., the nostalgia for the past, the quest for religious and political absolutes, the search for family stability and social order, the frightened call to return "back to the basics," and the like, percolate into the clinical relationship as well. Culture crisis creates the demand for authority to wrest order from chaos: the danger is that clinicians and politicians alike "comply"—for reasons of their own—with new rigidities borne more of anxiety than of comprehension.

Our conventional understandings of therapy, healing, cure, and the like—as much from within anthropology as within orthodox biomedicine—holds that disease or pathology is a departure or deviation from the social norm and that the goal of treatment is to restore the individual (insofar as it is possible) to the condition prior to falling ill (premorbid) and return him/her to society. Here, both the sanctity of the social norm and its supposed existence above the process that led to pathology in the first place are accepted uncritically. Yet, both theoretically and clinically, this position is incorrect, for the norm, the deviation from it, and the treatment alike are all part of the same social system (Mead 1947). Culturally, the goal of treatment is to change symptoms that a society's members as a whole *dislike*, which make them anxious, and to replace them with symptoms that its members *like* and that make them feel *reassured.* Cultural treatment is thus often symptom substitution.

Genuine therapy, on the other hand, is metacultural. That is, it is a form of *inner liberation,* not *social conformism,* for its aim is to help those who suffer to know their suffering, not simply to help them to find relief ("feel good," remission) from it. Genuine therapy identifies and ultimately gives the patient the courage to challenge the frightened, unthinking consensus that has often contributed to and culminated in the pathology. I define bona fide therapy as breaking the vicious cycle of pathology that includes one's defenses and symptoms. Therapy includes as well a deeper understanding of the conditions that produced these symptoms and how one unwittingly conspired with those circumstances. *Therapy* in this usage of the term is synonymous with inner liberation.

Our cultural definitions of therapy, however, have led us to embrace greater and greater specialization and the creation of a widening cornucopia of "units" of care. The proposed role of "*the* family" in family medicine is only the latest in this unfolding. Yet even this purported solution may share in the problem of the fragmentation of medicine and life. For the proper antidote to specialization is, not more specialization, but contextualization. What Sander writes of Jay Haley's strategic family therapy could well apply to much of the biomedical clinician's worldview that the family therapy movement, ideologically at least, repudiates: Many family therapy techniques

> sound like attempts to outsmart the patient and terminate the contract as quickly as possible. This approach leaves unanswered the question of how long-lasting the changes brought about will be and what the bases of these changes are. . . . The family systems paradigm assumes that significant portions of human behavior and experiences are (to degrees never fully realized) overdetermined by the social field and has demonstrated that as a modality it too can achieve symptomatic improvement. But to embrace behavioral change as a raison d'etre of family therapy will doom its further development. (Sander 1979:185)

The place where we must begin to break the vicious cycle of repetition lies, not in patient care, but in ourselves, practitioners, teachers, and administrators in medicine.

Patients are always trying to tell us something through their symptoms, diseases, resistances. They are trying to tell us their inner story even when they disguise it and "present" us only with the symptoms they feel safe enough to disclose. They are trying to tell us something even in the act of trying not to say something. Nurnberg and Shapiro, for instance, offer the concept of a "central organizing fantasy" (1983) as an assessment tool that can help orient the clinician to the clinical situation. Not only can we understand how people become ill from the way they form their fantasies but, "If the meaning an individual gives to his life and experiences has bearing on what makes him sick in the first place, it would seem that an effort to understand the dominant fantasy can offer an important insight into patients" (Nurnberg and Shapiro 1983:494–95).

We highly pragmatic, empirically minded Americans are so entirely attuned to happenings in the external world that in attempting to explain illness etiology, we concentrate almost exclusively on precipitants if not causes in the form of events rather than meanings. One thinks immediately of the Holmes and Rahe (1967) "Social Readjustment Rating Scale," for instance. However, "An event becomes a trauma and results in symptoms because of the unique meaning of the event to the affected individual" (Nurnberg and Shapiro 1983:494). It is as important to unravel the complex inner meaning of "what happened" as it is to uncover the often repressed and veiled experience of precisely what did happen.

So often in conducting a history, physical exam, and laboratory work-up, physicians are so eager to piece together their own story about what is wrong with the patient (which is important to do) that they unwittingly neglect to elicit the patient's own story—one that usually can be pieced together only over many episodes with individuals and combinations of family members. Developmentally, an organizing fantasy "refers to what the patient might say if he had full access to what is ordinarily unconscious, about the way he tends to see himself and his world, how this view developed out of his experience, and how it influences his behavior and his fears" (Nurnberg and Shapiro 1983:497). If medicine is truly to be meaning-centered (Good and Good 1981), the physician must become better aware of those meanings that he/she brings to the clinical encounter, those meanings brought by the patient, how one perceives and feels about the patient, and therefore what one wishes to see and not to see in the patient. Only by gaining greater familiarity with one's own personal and professional story can one become increasingly adept at eliciting and hearing the inner story that the patient and family is trying to tell the physician through the symptoms and history.

Child psychiatrist Alice Miller writes that: "It is a fascinating experience to accompany a patient on this journey [of discovery]— so long as we do not try to enter this new land with concepts that are familiar to us, perhaps in order to avoid our own fear of what is unknown and not yet understood. The patient discovers his true self little by little through experiencing his own feelings and needs, because the analyst is able to accept and respect these even when he does not yet understand them" (1981:76–77). I see no reason why learning to embark on this journey should not constitute part of the professional training of all physicians. If we as medical educators offer future providers only socially approved defenses, we shall succeed only in rendering virtually inaccessible not only the inner pain of the practitioner to himself or herself but that of the patient as well. In the guise of maintaining a therapeutic position, one will be deaf and mute to deeper stirrings that can thus only be acted out as defenses.

"The psychiatrist," writes La Barre, "must know himself, through a rigorous and often painful didactic analysis, for he will not be able to see in his patients what he cannot afford to see in terms of his own defenses. He must constantly ask 'What am I doing in saying this or asking that?'—that is, he must carefully watch his own countertrans-ference to the patient" (1978:269). Lamentably, such disciplined self-awareness is not only no longer an inexorable part of psychiatric training, it is virtually absent from biomedical training. Thus, for the most part, even behavioral scientists direct all their—and medical students' and residents'—attention to the patients', and now the families', behavior and studiously avoid inner meanings of behavior in themselves, in patients and families, and in those whom they are teaching. We search for formulas about ethnic behavior and family interaction as eagerly as physicians rely on formulas about the efficacy of mastectomy and antibiotics.

Yet, for physician and behavioral scientist alike, to peer inward is an invaluable—nay, an essential—tool for looking outward. One can be therapeutic—irrespective of the name of one's specialty— only as one is capable of hearing and feeling what the patient is trying to say or not to say. We must be capable of being moved by the patient and aware of precisely how we are moved. Observing the outside alone can function as a profoundly powerful defense against looking within—and thereby distorting what is outside as well. The question of whether to order this test, to do that pro-cedure, or to interpret some result in one way rather than another must always be partly answered in terms of what we do so *for* in terms of our unconscious meaning. The unexamined life is one that observes and interprets what to a large degree it first projected.

In his still revolutionary essay "The Golden Rule in the Light of New Insight," Erik Erikson defined mutuality to be "a relationship in which partners depend on each other for the development of their respective strengths" (1964:231). He then proceeds to reformulate the Golden Rule in the light of a psychoanalytic understanding of human development: *"truly worthwhile acts enhance a mutuality between the doer and the other—a mutuality which strengthens the doer even as it strengthens the other* (1964:233). Erikson then specifies "a mutuality of divided function, . . . a professional, and yet relatively intimate, one: that between healer and patient" (1964:236), which "permits the medical man to *develop as a practitioner, and as a person, even as the patient is cured as a patient, and as a person"* (1964:236). *One is thus most capable of being therapeutic*—responding to the depth of the patient—not when one writes oneself out of the clinical equation (for no sooner does one dissociate one's personal self from the clinical situation than one makes the patient likewise into an inanimate object), but *when one can recognize that one is always a part of the clinical equation.*

REFERENCES

Balint, M. 1957. *The doctor, his patient, and the illness.* New York: International Universities Press.

Bateson, G. 1972. *Steps to an ecology of mind: Collected essays in anthropology, psychiatry, evolution, and epistemology.* San Francisco: Chandler.

Boyer, L. B. 1983. Approaching cross-cultural psychotherapy. *The Journal of Psychoanalytic Anthropology* 6(3):237–45.

Buber, M. 1958. *I and thou,* 2d ed., translated by R. G. Smith. New York: Charles Scribner's Sons (orig. 1923).

———. 1965. Dialogue, translated by R. G. Smith. In *Between man and man.* New York: Macmillan.

Candib, L. M. 1987. What doctors tell about themselves to patients: Implications for intimacy and reciprocity in the relationship. *Family Medicine* 19(1):23–30.

Devereux, G. 1980. Normal and abnormal. In his *Basic problems of ethnopsychiatry,* translated by B. M. Gulati and G. Devereux, 3–71. Chicago: University of Chicago Press (orig. 1956).

———. 1967. *From anxiety to method in the behavioral sciences.* The Hague: Mouton.

Draguns, J. G. 1981. Cross-cultural counseling and psychotherapy: History, issues, and current status. In *Cross-cultural counseling and psychotherapy,* edited by A. Marsella and P. Pedersen. Elmsford, N.Y.: Pergamon.

Erikson, E. H. 1964. The golden rule in the light of new insight. In his *Insight and responsibility,* 219–43. New York: Norton.

Freud, S. 1910. The future prospects of psycho-analytic therapy. In *The standard edition of the complete psychological works of Sigmund Freud (SE)* 11, translated by J. Strachey, 139–51. London: Hogarth Press, 1957.

———. 1914. Observations on transference-love. *SE* 12, translated by J. Strachey, 157–71. London: Hogarth Press, 1958.

Good, B. J., and M. D. Good. 1981. The meaning of symptoms: A cultural hermeneutic model for clinical practice. In *The relevance of social science for medicine,* edited by L. Eisenberg and A. Kleinman, 165–96. Dordrecht, Holland: D. Reidel.

Gutheil, T. G., H. Bursztajn, and A. Brodsky. 1984. Sounding board: Malpractice prevention through the sharing of uncertainty. *The New England Journal of Medicine* 311:49–51.

Holmes, T. H., and R. H. Rahe. 1967. The social readjustment rating scale. *The Journal of Psychosomatic Research* 11:213–18.

Kerenyi, C. 1959. *Asklepios: Archetypal image of the physician's existence,* Bollingen Series, vol. 3. Princeton, N.J.: Princeton University Press.

Kiefer, C. W. 1976. Review of *Morita-Psychotherapy* by D. Reynolds. *Medical Anthropology Newsletter* 7(4):11–12.

Kleinman, A. 1980. *Patients and healers in the context of culture: An exploration of the borderland between anthropology, medicine, and psychiatry.* Berkeley and Los Angeles: University of California Press.

Kluckhohn, F., and F. Strodtbeck. 1961. *Variations in value orientations.* Evanston, Ill.: Row Peterson.

La Barre, W. 1975. Anthropological perspectives on hallucination and hallucinogens. In *Hallucinations: Behavior, experience, and theory,* edited by R. K. Siegel and L. J. West, 9–52. New York: Wiley.

———. 1978. The clinic and the field. In *The making of psychological anthropology,* edited by G. D. Spindler, 258–99. Berkeley and Los Angeles: University of California Press.

Langs, R. 1978. *Technique in transition.* New York: Jason Aronson.

Mead, M. 1947. The concept of culture and the psychosomatic approach. *Psychiatry* 10:57–76.

Miller, A. 1981. *The drama of the gifted child: How narcissistic parents form and deform the emotional lives of their talented children,* translated by R. Ward. New York: Basic Books (orig. 1979).

Modell, A. 1976. "The holding environment" and the therapeutic action of psychoanalysis. *The Journal of the American Psychoanalytic Association* 24: 285–307.

Nurnberg, H. G., and L. M. Shapiro. 1983. The central organizing fantasy. *Psychoanalytic Review* 70(4):493–503.

Olinick, S. L. 1969. On empathy and regression in the service of the other. *British Journal of Medical Psychology* 42:41–49.

Opler, M. 1936. Some points of comparison and contrast between the treatment of functional disorders by Apache shamans and modern psychiatric practice. *American Journal of Psychiatry* 92:1371–87.

Pellegrino, E., and D. Thomasma. 1982. *The philosophical basis of medical practice.* New York: Oxford University Press.

Sander, F. M. 1979. *Individual and family therapy: Toward an integration.* New York: Jason Aronson.

Searles, H. F. 1975. The patient as therapist to his analyst. In *Tactics and techniques in psychoanalytic therapy*, vol. 2, *Countertransference*, edited by P. L. Giovacchini, 95–151. New York: Jason Aronson.

Smith, R. C., and H. F. Stein. 1987. A topographical model of clinical decision making and interviewing. *Family Medicine* 19(5):361–63.

Spiegel, J. 1971. *Transactions: The interplay between individual, family, and society.* New York: Science House.

Stein, H. F., and R. F. Hill. 1977. *The ethnic imperative: Examining the new white ethnic movement.* University Park: Pennsylvania State University Press.

Stephens, G. G. 1984. What's true about what's new? Manuscript, The Blanchard Lecture, Society of Teachers of Family Medicine, Orlando, Florida, May 7.

Volkan, V. D. 1981. Transference and countertransference: An examination from the point of view of internalized object relations. In *Object and self: A developmental approach*, edited by S. Tuttman, C. Kaye, and M. Zimmerman, 429–51. New York: International Universities Press.

Wintrob, R. 1973. The influence of others: Witchcraft and rootwork as explanation of behavior disturbances. *The Journal of Nervous and Mental Disorders* 156:318–26.

CHAPTER 2

Where is "The Case"?
A Psychoanalytic-Ethnographic
Inquiry into the Boundary of
Pathology in a
Spinal Cord-Injured Woman

HOWARD F. STEIN

INTRODUCTION

The concept of a case is, from the viewpoints of assessment, diagnosis, treatment, and outcome—in any society—intrinsically bound up with multiple conceptions or constructions of the boundary of what and who are included and excluded. To oversimplify: a classical psychoanalytic case focuses on the analysand's mental life; a classical biomedical physician is for the most part concerned with a diseased organ and its repair; countless preliterate societies assemble entire extended families, even communities of contiguous kin and nonkin, to ritually remove the collective poison and restore community health and well-being. This chapter documents an attempt to trace out, so to speak, the network of relationships and meanings involved in the refractory depression of a woman injured in an automobile accident some years ago. It will incidentally further validate Dundes's hypothesis (1985) that the basis for depth-psychology interpretations lies within the very materials of the culture.

This study describes the course of ethnographically informed counseling with a woman who had sustained a spinal-cord injury in an automobile accident that left her right side seriously impaired. It offers a perspective on how one might integrate, both conceptually and in clinical practice, such seemingly disparate realms as the patient's intrapsychic domain, her family of origin, interaction in her current family (including both the family of origin and the family of procreation), her religious and other cultural belief system and church membership, her life in a small, rural Oklahoma farming town (population 1,000), and her multiple relationships with health-care personnel. The unfolding of counseling reveals that the intrapsychic, interactional, and cultural realms can all be understood to be perspectives of a central dynamic. This core structure includes, but is not limited to, the patient or symptom-bearer: namely, it is the role played by the unconscious in organizing personalities, families, groups, communities, and "whole" cultures. Peoples' fantasies about themselves and others will be seen to function as an integrative process and structure, so that in order to complete the patient's conscious and intrapsychic story, his or her social "reality" must be analyzable (Devereux 1980)—for that is part of the patient as he/she is part of it.

Winter in the southern Great Plains of North America is plagued with treacherous ice storms that coat every exposed surface with a layer of ice. It was in the wake of one such storm that the patient, whom I shall refer to as Carol, sustained her spinal-cord injury. She was a passenger in the front seat of a friend's car and was not wearing a seat belt. Enough of the road had begun to clear that drivers acted upon the false security of dry pavement. Car speeds accelerated from the cautious crawl to the presumptuous. The car in which Carol was riding suddenly hit a patch of ice on the road, spun, and turned over several times, throwing Carol and the driver around the interior. Almost miraculously, the driver walked away without injury. Carol's life was changed.

In the accident Carol injured the brachial plexus of her cervical spine region, permanently damaging her right upper and lower extremities. Her discharge diagnoses were: Cervical fracture dislocation of C5 and C6 treated orthopedically and in immobilization; and Brown-Sequard syndrome (spinal hemiplegia). In the months following the nearly fatal accident, Carol had great determination in her physical therapy. She had hoped to restore all the functions she had lost in her right arm and leg. She was walking and using her right hand in daily homemaking activities. Carol gained strength far more quickly than any of the health professionals had anticipated. At the same time, she could not completely recover all the subtle movements and strength she had previously possessed. Her nine-year-old son persistently urged her to do push-ups! Her husband, children, and community at the Baptist church expected her to "get back to normal." They avoided bringing up the subject of her lingering disability—or at least acknowledging her real limitations. Their fantasies about her and expectations of her became a burden on her, and became woven into her own intrapsychic world of anticipated recovery and utter independence. Over the course of therapy, her sense of having and being a distinct self tenuously began to emerge from her complex unconscious social web of obligations as a standard-bearer for others.

When a serious illness or disability strikes a person and, in turn, his or her family and wider social network (occupational, church, etc.), a clinician ideally asks two types of questions: (1) In a lineal or Newtonian sense, how does a disease or disability affect a change in a person and his/her milieu? (2) In a systems or circular sense, how is a disease or disability incorporated into the meaning and relationship structure of a person, family, and group? For instance, Carol had felt that prior to the auto accident, she could at least control her own body, when she could scarcely control her children. Following the accident, she felt deprived even of this bastion of effectiveness. She wished to be a staunchly independent person, yet felt throttled in her efforts by her accident and disability.

At the same time, she had never learned to drive a car—a fact she long blamed on the failure of others to teach her, and only recently has she acknowledged her own fearfulness to learn to drive. Unable to gain control over her own life and body as completely as she wished after the accident, Carol watched and noticed intensely the independence, if not defiance, exhibited by her children and husband. What she now lacked and felt deprived of, she contended with and scrutinized both enviously and resentfully in them. Much of the time in therapy was spent discussing problems that antedated the accident, problems that the accident intensified but did not cause. The better I came to know her, the more I realized how Carol's, her family's, and her community's adaptation to the disability was a new variation on an old theme.

CONTEXT OF MY INVOLVEMENT IN THE CASE

When the clinician closes the door to the examining room or the consultation or family-therapy room, one often harbors the fiction that he or she is alone with the patient or the family and can proceed with therapy. To avoid creating this illusion in this case study, it is best that I identify from the outset the dramatis personae (including the institutions) whose presence loomed large over the course of the year and a half of psychotherapy. The patient, Carol, (thirty-eight at the beginning of treatment) was married to a ma-

chinist who worked at a foundry in a medium-size Oklahoma crossroads town some twenty miles from their home in a rural farming
town. They had two children, a son age nine and a daughter age
four at the beginning of therapy. They were members of a Baptist
church in their town, a church and community that prided itself on
knowing everything about everyone while officially prizing family
privacy. The patient's mother-in-law, who lived in their town, drove
the patient to medical visits (etc.) when her husband could not do so.

I first saw Carol eight months after the automobile accident in
which she had been a passenger. After her hospitalization in a
distant medical complex, she had been referred for follow-up and
continuity of care to a family physician in Crossroads, a larger town
twenty miles from her home. That family physician in turn coordinated her care with a physical therapist at a local community hospital. He also asked me to work with her on her psychosocial adjustment (he had diagnosed her as having situational depression). He
arranged to continue seeing her at the family medicine clinic in
Crossroads (where I also worked one day each week) to monitor her
physical rehabilitation and treat any physical complaints. I worked
closely with him, providing him verbal as well as typewritten sum-
maries following each session. We regularly discussed her progress
and agreed on how to proceed. Following early sessions, I also
discussed the case with her referring physician and psychotherapist
(of the "strategic" school) at the distant medical complex (with
which I was also affiliated). She had been scheduled to return there
at lengthening intervals for follow-up and progress assessment as
well. Although I could have attempted to proceed with Carol on
an exclusively—and illusory—one-to-one basis, I elected to work
closely with her entire treatment context as part of my work with
her.

The final contexts I wish to identify in setting the stage for the
case discussion are those labeled by Devereux (1969, 1978:403–4,
1980) as cross-cultural (or intercultural) and transcultural (or meta-
cultural) therapy. The term *cross-cultural* refers to the fact that the
patient and I were from different cultures, and that I took her
cultural belief and value system into account during the course of
therapy. The term *transcultural* refers to the fact that the goal of
therapy is beyond the framework of the cultural system that is at
least in part responsible for the patient's symptoms and predica-
ment in the first place. Transcultural therapy may use cultural
materials to accomplish its goal (Devereux 1969), but it does not
treat them as "givens" not to be examined in terms of their psycho-

logical functions and meanings for the patient, family, and larger group (see also Stein 1985e).

Carol and her family and community were rural, Baptist, Oklahomans, while I was from a mill town near Pittsburgh, Pennsylvania, and of Jewish origins. Many Oklahomans have referred to those from "Back East" as DamnYankees (which, I am told, can be construed as a single noun). With my cultural and professional past, I had become relatively comfortable with exploring with others the meaning of their dreams. I quickly learned from many white Christian Oklahomans—farmers, physicians, medical students, patients—that dreams were a virtually taboo topic to broach, for many people feared that the interlocutor might know too much too soon about them and subsequently condemn them. They feared their dreams and their potential meanings, often dreading that to recall a dream or to have it interpreted would reveal that they were "crazy," "abnormal," "sinful," or "evil," or that even their own thoughts were "out of control."

Although Carol, her family and community, and I shared ostensibly the same American language, the therapy was, of necessity, a bona fide cross-cultural experience: I had to be careful not to make any assumptions about shared symbols, shared meanings, or even shared expectations about what constituted "therapy." I had hoped, for instance, to have husband and wife participate in at least a few sessions together (to discuss and evaluate their changed relationship as a result of her disability and their problems in child rearing). The husband attended only once, and even then he kept his active participation to a minimum. As I have noted elsewhere (Stein 1985d, 1985e), whereas many white Oklahoman rural women will discuss personal and family problems with their family doctor or pastor, white Oklahoman men generally do not wish to acknowledge the existence of personal or family problems. They often feel that there are no problems they cannot—and should not—handle themselves within the privacy of their home, or by flight from their home into work in the fields, pasturelands, machine shop, or oil rig. To them, the idea of assembling a married couple, or a whole family, for the purpose of discussing a problem with a nonfamily member is either repugnant or unnecessary. To me, on the other hand, the notion of conducting family therapy by seeing an individual family member was less a matter of doctrinal or conceptual integrity (e.g., Bowen 1978) than it was the only culturally acceptable modality.

This brings me to a broader "methodological"—in fact, contextual—point: as therapists, physicians, applied anthropologists, and the like, we are always working with and within other people's systems of meanings and structures. Perhaps to be most respectful—and thereby most effective—we should take those systems seriously into account and not try to insist that the only context that matters in therapy is our own! In a recent paper in family-systems therapy with an individual, McHolland says in very undoctrinaire fashion that "Family-systems theory is applicable not only for families or other systems but also for individual clients as well. Many individuals still come *alone* for counseling and therapy. They do not bring their families. Their families won't come or they don't want them to. . . . Does that mean we cannot provide a systems-oriented individual therapy? I think not. Whether we acknowledge it or not, every individual really *does* bring the various systems in which one is involved at least to some degree" (1985:62–63).

REPLAYING FAMILY-OF-ORIGIN ISSUES

From the family physician's description of the patient, I had imagined and expected therapy to center around the feelings of loss and sadness associated with her spinal-cord injury. I was wrong. Carol spent many sessions fighting any sense of loss or grief (as I realized only later in therapy) *by* fighting with her children. Session 5, for instance, began as many had begun previously, and as many later ones were to begin: with a litany of complaints about her children's misbehavior: "My son's louder than ever. He's constantly aggravating me. He aggravates his sister just to hear her scream. He just won't listen."

In previous sessions, I had responded literally to the disciplining problem, and discussed with Carol (and once with both her and her husband) a strategy of checking with each other when setting limits on the son's behavior so that he could not play one off against the other. I soon came to feel that such a response was a trap, for it would keep our focus on their son. As she spoke this time, I found myself wondering what *she* had been like when she was eight or nine years old. She was talking about her son, but as I experienced her, I visualized her as her son. I responded with this fantasy and asked her to tell what she recalled about herself and her family when she was her son's age.

> Mom gave me the broom [hit her with the broom] when I mouthed. I got more discipline from Mom than from Dad. When I'd talk back, I got

hit in the mouth. I didn't like it, but I've come to realize that I deserved it. [I asked her about how many siblings she had, her place in the sibling order, etc.] There were eight of us growing up. Mom would make us mind. I'm the sixth, with a younger brother and sister. Mom said I was a good kid. Although I had a mouth too, like our son, from when I was four to when I was twelve I had seizures, then at twelve they diagnosed them, and brought them under control. Mom didn't discipline me much. She was afraid of hurting me because of the seizures. . . . When I was twelve or so, my sister and I ran away—for two hours [laugh]! We walked two miles, took cigarettes and an overnight blanket. We didn't get our way at home, so we left. Mom came after us, and said that we walked that far, and we could walk back home!

I offered the interpretation that she and her son identified with one another, and that it might have been difficult for her to learn to control herself consistently when, on the one hand, her mother sometimes would hit her, and on the other hand, her mother would let her get away with things because she was afraid of harming her. In this session and others, we spent much time talking about how difficult it was for her to hold herself back from hitting her son, yet how the things that most angered her about him, were also some of her own—sometimes disliked, sometimes proudly held—qualities. She continued:

My son and I are both strong willed and opinionated. That's why I've got to get him while he's still young and opinionated [she said adamantly]. He brings homework home instead of finishing it in school. The teacher tells him that he could finish it in school and not have to bring it home. I try to back her up, and tell him that if he finished it at school, he'd be able to play with his friends. I'd like him to learn responsibility. He leaves his shoes and dirty clothes on the floor, can't find them. My husband is the same way. I've always felt responsible. You've got to mold them, or they won't turn out responsible.

I made an interpretation that she seemed to be locked in a vicious cycle of responsibility and resentment and rebellion, and was identifying with her son's behavior. I also thought, but did not interpret, her considerable closeness with her son that was both expressed and given distance by their frequent fighting. I felt that Oedipal/Jocasta–level interpretations, even if correct, would be ill-timed, and either rejected outright or felt as overwhelmingly shame-inducing. (My experience with rural whites in the American Great Plains culture area has been that what might be offered as an

interpretation, even speculation, by the therapist aimed at problem
solving can often be experienced as a horrible accusation that either
must not be true or is oppressively valid—the latter leading to
defensive countershaming maneuvers.) Over time—as I learned
not to be lured into futile advice-giving—I redirected her exasperation with her son (or daughter, or husband) to an examination of
her own feelings and their source in her own family past; even more
gradually did we both come to realize that the steadfastness of her
preoccupation with her family's lack of control was a metaphor for
her own feelings of loss and helplessness in the face of the auto
accident. Unable to grieve for what she had—perhaps permanently—lost, she railed and thundered about what those did who
possessed the energy and mobility she no longer had.

The patient is Seminole and English on both parents' side of the
family. Both grandfathers were Baptist preachers, although she
and her seven siblings were reared in an almost defiantly irreli-
gious household. Carol said that her father, long divorced from
her mother—yet remarried and living across the street from her
mother—had had a conversion experience and became a Christian
several years ago. She lamented that her mother was not a Christian, that is, had failed to have the experience of being born again.
Carol, her husband, and their two children regularly attended the
Baptist church in their town, and she said that she would like to be
Christian (which is not synonymous with church membership and
participation).

From my experience with patients and nonpatients in this region, I contend that Carol's *vacillation between defiance and obedience,*
and its representation in religious symbolism (especially that of
evangelical Protestantism), is a widespread personal, family, and
cultural theme (Stein 1987b; see also LaBarre 1972). Families officially pride themselves on their conformity; they tell me of the
preachers, the upstanding farmers, the "family" men and women
who uphold the community standard. But with a twinkle and a note
of condemnation that fuses boastfulness with embarrassment, they
tell me likewise of an uncle, or aunt, or grandparent who was
hanged as a horse thief or cattle rustler, or who made a bundle
through gambling and then lost it all, or who married and left
behind a string of spouses. Religion is a hoped-for source of exte-
rior control that must be found and rebelled against, since that
control is so lacking from within. Stated otherwise, conflict is more
often experienced externally than internally; it is experienced and

represented in various family and community roles rather than, for the most part, in facets of oneself.[1]

Thus, it was a major achievement for Carol over the course of counseling to begin to acknowledge that she was herself something of a rebel in addition to prizing order and independence in her life. She grudgingly came to realize that she not only resented her husband's and children's disruptive and provocative behavior but that they were acting that way at her behest. She, in turn, tried unsuccessfully and ambivalently to set limits on them (as Kohutian "self-objects," see Kohut 1971).

CONTROL, PERFECTION, AND THE DREAD OF FAILURE

The auto accident and its aftermath stretched Carol's values to the breaking point; her values then exacted from her more than she could physically give. She took herself severely to task for not being able to restore herself to perfection—to walk well, to carry even the heaviest casserole, to be a good enough wife, mother, and Christian.[2]

---

[1]In a brilliant and controversial essay on "The Evolution of Childhood," psycho-historian deMause (1974) characterized what he terms the "intrusive mode" or style of child rearing. His description fits my own observations among rural "white" Great Plains farming families from a variety of ancestral ethnic groups: e.g., German, Czech, English, Scotch-Irish, Polish, groups that over the generations forged a common "culture area" and "areal ethos" (see Devereux 1969; Kroeber 1930; Stein 1987b) that has become a regional hallmark (see Stein 1985c). Irrespective of the reader's agreement with deMause's evolutionary scheme, his description is apt for Carol and her "object world": "parents . . . attempted to conquer [the child's] mind, in order to control its insides, its anger, its needs, its masturbation, its very will. The child raised by intrusive parents was nursed by the mother, not swaddled, not given regular enemas [although especially in older German families in the region, enemas for children and among adults alike were a still familiar mode of purging: HFS], toilet trained early, prayed with but not played with, hit but not regularly whipped, punished for masturbation, and made to obey promptly with threats and guilt as often as with other methods of punishment" (1974:52). During economic depressions and cultural panics in the region, there occurs a similar regression to earlier, more primitive child rearing: e.g., frequent beatings to rid the child of evil—together with collective reaction formations (revulsion, outrage) and campaigns against child abuse; and the obsession with molding the child into shape, out of fear that the child would become wild and evil (deMause 1974:51).

[2]A Southern Baptist family physician colleague, who has counseled many ministerial couples and served as their family doctor, tells me of one Baptist minister's wife whom he had treated for multiple physical complaints, none of which could be attributed to an organic disease process. When he offered to her the interpretation that the symptoms might be stress related, she adamantly replied: "I am a Christian, I *can't* have stress"—a statement that the physician, I believe accurately, construed as meaning that as she expected herself and her marriage to be perfect, any flaw in that perfection must be

What Carol could not compel from herself, she tried strenuously to compel from her children and she keenly felt compelled by her religious community and family. Living in a community that could be widely described in terms of what deMause (1974) calls the "intrusive mode" of child rearing, she possessed a persecutory, incompletely internalized superego. As I worked with her, I keenly felt her sense of shame to be far more paramount than a sense of guilt for wrongdoings or wrong thoughts.

For a while, I found it maddeningly difficult to *locate* where all her conscience was, for it did not feel as if it were installed inside her. Sometimes she would be her own unforgiving judge. At other times, her children, or husband, would be her impulsive self, and she would be the enraged parents avenging themselves for righteousness sake. At still other times, she would be the victim of her moral community—her family, church, town, all expecting her to recover fully on her own, offering no succor or aid. It felt to me as if a complex system of self, family, church, and community was "fueled" by an interlocking network of externalization and projective identification from which there was no exit. In fact, to wish to exit would signify one's immorality in the eyes of the community and of God as well. (Technically speaking, her conflicts were more object-relations type than classical structural theory type.)

In Carol's Baptist world, self-control was prized; if she had lost it through the accident, she would regain it—by herself. It was a test: if she regained complete use of her hand, arm, and leg, it would be proof that she was worthy; if she failed, it would show to all that she was a failure. She felt very much alone in her attempts at recovery— and in her attempts at differentiating between what were realistic goals and what were magical ones. Her slow "hatching"—if I may borrow a term from Margaret Mahler, who developed it with reference to an infant hatching from a mother-child symbiosis (Mahler and Furer 1968)—from the family and community symbiosis was an awesome experience for me to witness. By the end of therapy, her realization of the *difference* between her expectations and her reality was a herculean accomplishment, one that permitted her finally to begin to mourn her loss rather than only to rage against it and try to undo it through others.

Carol's fear of failure dominated many sessions. The eighth

---

denied. Carol's self-blame, and its association with evangelical Protestant religious values, is not idiosyncratic or isolated, but characterizes many born-again Christians and those seeking or awaiting spiritual rebirth.

session, for instance, began with her relating an incident that had occurred at home just prior to the session. She had been in a hurry to leave for the appointment. Her four-year-old daughter was eating breakfast very slowly. Carol finally became so angry with her daughter's "delay tactics," that she "took the switch to her"—and now felt guilty. She talked about the fact that she loves her children, but doesn't like them all the time. She feared that the distinction was a sign that she was "crazy," and that I would condemn her for being a bad mother. In her personal, family, and community world, liking and loving were fused. Imperfect love, such as disliking some aspects of one whom you love, was not tolerated; it was regarded as un-Christian. It was considered to be a sign of one's deep flaw and failure in the many eyes that stretch along one's path from oneself to God. "Most people won't admit they don't like their kids. I don't like their attitude. Because I think there are times that everybody doesn't especially like the attitude or behavior of someone who they love." It took much trust and courage for her to say what others in her family, church, and town could not—must not—admit to ever *thinking*. No sooner did she express negative feelings toward her children, than she came down hard on herself once again, as if to punish herself for daring to acknowledge anger toward those whom one was expected to love perfectly. She became tearful: "I really believe that I don't like myself. The way I am, my physical condition, I can't control my temper. No control. I do my therapy every day, but I'm not making good progress. I'm trying hard, but I feel like a failure even though the doctors and you all say how well I'm doing. I've been tempted to try doing push-ups to see whether I could do them [her son had been taunting her about doing push-ups], but I think I could harm my hand or shoulder even more than they are now. I feel like a failure. If I liked myself I'd not feel depressed and unhappy." As she was talking, I wondered why the sense of failure was especially poignant then. I did not want to fall into the trap of trying to find advice or recipes for her happiness. I fantasized aloud that I wondered whether her approaching fortieth birthday, a major life landmark in Judeo-Christian society, had anything to do with her sense of urgency—and therefore with her harshness toward her daughter (since the issue of not enough time was most pressing in their struggle of wills). At first she smiled a glance of recognition, then became tearful:

I don't drive [a car]. I want to be a success at something, but I haven't found anything I can do successfully. I don't like to think about getting old. My accomplishments don't measure up to my goals. I always wanted to be a nurse. I was the only one of eight children to graduate from high school. I really stuck with it to get there. In the first place I wanted to be an R.N., but I didn't think I was smart enough to be one, so I took the L.P.N., the easy way out. I worked as [an] L.P.N. fifteen months at the hospital. Then I married my husband. He didn't want me to work. I worked a few times at the extended-care center in my town, but then I just stayed away. I try to do whatever the good Lord wants. I always felt a failure in spending all that money and time to go to school, and then came the accident. I read the newspaper, and read all the ads; I'm looking for something I can do. I need to drive or have more skills. But [bitterly], I am successful only in my therapy. [Earlier in the session, she had felt herself to be a failure even in therapy. Here, I think that she was bitterly protesting that only in the patient role, which she consciously despised, was she even remotely good at anything. HFS]

I felt pulled to try to rescue her from her sense of futility and despair; I despaired that anything I might say could be reassuring. "I can't take your sense of despair away from you. You have gone through a lot." I wanted to acknowledge, confirm, the reality of her loss and not contribute to her evading it. At the same time, I wanted to assess the social and occupational realities she had available, and her response to their availability or lack. We had talked a number of times about her considering taking driving lessons from a local school for handicapped drivers. I asked her whether she had checked the local school. She replied that school had just started that week, in fact, but that she had forgotten to check. She added that she had thought of applying for a position as teacher's aide, but feared that she could go only in good weather. "What's holding me back? [she asked tearfully] Fear? Fear of failure?" We talked further of her tendency to couch everything in either/or, black/white, terms: that she would either be a total success or an utter failure at learning to drive. I wondered aloud whether she could approach driving, vocational training, etc., more in a spirit of playfulness or experimentation. This might help her to get out of the vicious cycle of fearing failure, of needing to be in total control, and of avoiding doing things that threaten her loss of control. Her eyes brightened, as if she had never permitted herself to entertain such a thought before. "Maybe there's something more to life than dreading failure. I've never thought about that."

THE RECURRENT DREAM

Almost exactly a year after the accident, during session 5, I asked Carol how she was feeling as the anniversary of the accident approached. First angrily, then tearfully, she said: "I should have made more progress. I want my hand to be back to normal. It'll never be back to normal. When I put on my clothes, necklace, earrings—I have pierced ears—I can't do them all myself. When I get nervous, I can't button my jeans. *Restrictions*, that's what I dislike so much. I don't like to be like this. I can't carry heavy casseroles myself, but I've got to ask for help. When somebody helps me, it makes me mad. I have no patience. I can't stand to wait." Her family, too, I had learned, was equally impatient; and her family and church community had difficulty continuing to acknowledge her *need* for help. I might add that, in marked contrast with this apparent collective and accumulative denial of Carol's disability, it is a widespread cultural gesture as well as value in this Great Plains region to offer an immediate, short-term assistance of some kind *behaviorally* (such as helping with cooking, bringing food, gathering to build a barn, etc.) instead of verbally, as soon as family or friends notice that some sort of assistance is needed: that is, to offer help without ever being asked, to help those receiving aid be able to save face by not requiring them to ask for it. The discrepancy between the cultural rule of how to act toward "normals" and her community's behavior toward her—a deviant—was bitterly clear to her. She could now no longer expect what others could take for granted.

As she was speaking about her entire family's monumental impatience and impulsivity, it suddenly flashed through my mind why—perhaps—her son's misbehavior had recently been such an object of her fascination and resentment. As she finished talking about her inability to accept limitations upon her capacities, and her (as well as her parents') monumental impatience, I said to her: "Could it be that your son is acting the way you'd like to act? You're seeing in him what you can't be now, and maybe never will be again?" She became tearful, replying, "I think that's it." We both began to understand what some of the deeper issues beneath the conscious struggle for controlling him were about: she had projected part of herself onto him. She continued: "My mother-in-law says to me 'Your hand ought to be back [to normal] in about a year.' She tells people at church, 'One of these days she'll be able to use it [her right hand] again.'" Just as we had discussed her projective identification onto her son, she in essence told me that she was the identical sort of target of magical projective thinking from her mother-in-law (and family and church).

Shortly after, Carol said pensively, while looking at her right hand (which she rarely did): "This may be the way I am." I said that she probably would be thinking often around this time of the year (the first anniversary) about her accident, maybe even having dreams about it. She said with a mixture of surprise and hesitation: "You mean that doesn't mean I'm losing my mind?" We discussed her association of dreams with being "crazy," "abnormal," and therefore outcast, an association widely shared among Oklahoma whites, especially those of fundamentalist Christian groups. I respected her fears, but said that from my viewpoint, dreaming was a normal human activity, and not a sign of madness. She then courageously recounted her recurrent dream: "I have dreams about my hand being normal, and that's disturbing to me because I wake up and it hasn't changed. I want my hand to be normal. Yet I know that might never happen. I wake up and I'm mad, because I see my hand perfect in my dream, then I see it as it really is."

Boundary issues in her family and community complicated her grieving and reintegrating process. Not only did she externalize her own conflicts over impulse control onto her children and husband, she was likewise their receptacle for their own difficulties in mourning. Her struggle to delineate a personal boundary (and a boundary between parent and spouse as well) was waged over the vicissitudes of her recovery from the automobile accident.

It was a major accomplishment for her to report during session 6 that several weeks earlier

> I told my husband that I wanted our daughter out of our bedroom. She slept there four years, first in her crib, then in her little bed. Two weeks ago we moved out her furniture, so that we could have more privacy. We gave her a special room, enough room for her forty dolls. Her room is now like a disaster area! [She said this with a sparkle of delight in her eyes, and a smile—which she often does when she complains of her children's misbehavior, which she also admires.] My husband and I never have time to ourselves. Our daughter first balked when we moved her. She was crying. So we left the big light on in her room; later we just left the little light on. Her crying diminished. So we now have our room to ourselves.

Later in session 6 she said: "Every so often I get upset. I don't want to be the center of attention, but I'd like people in my family to ask 'How are you doing?' People think that I should already be completely recuperated. Other people's lack of interest in how I'm progressing aggravates me. Especially my husband's."

We talked about the different rates of acceptance in her family of her degree of disability—which both compounded her own issues of acceptance and displaced her attention from an internal issue to criticizing their lack of acceptance. We also talked about the difference between people's experience of disability following an accident versus their experience of chronic illness: to her family, Carol had not been sick. Therefore, conferring on her the sick role for an extended period of time did not make sense. We also discussed her family's tendency and hers toward impatience and wanting to solve everything immediately (that is, their problem-solving style). I urged that she should be explicit with them about what is realistic for her and what her current limits are. I wondered whether she could feel free to test reality even if her family and community could not accept it as theirs. Here, I wanted to affirm her own nascent sense of boundaries and self, even if those close to her were insisting that she could do anything she wanted if she only applied herself. She then returned to discussion of her dreams: "What does the hand symbolize? [I asked her what she thought. Poignantly she replied, while holding her injured hand over her heart:] My head knows that it'll never be back to the way it was, but my heart wants it back the way it was. Up here [pointing to her head], I know it's hard to get better, like it was. My son just said to me: 'How come you're not doing push-ups? If you really tried, you could. . . .' He wants me back like I was. He cried while I was in the hospital." Her motility in assigning meanings and feelings first inside herself, then outside herself in her son (and others), could not be more clearly stated.

As counseling progressed, one of my chief tasks was to help Carol to hold onto conflicts long enough to experience them as her own rather than (exclusively) as originating with someone else. Stated more technically, her shared *object-relations style* of personal, family, and group representation and cohesion made her grieving especially difficult and protracted (see Volkan 1981). It also greatly limited my own leverage in therapy, since her family's blurring of personal boundaries was literally coextensive with the milieu in which she lived.

Although I shall discuss countertransference issues as a separate topic, I should say here that I experienced feelings of frustration, impatience, even exasperation as Carol recounted episode after episode of her efforts to control herself and her family, while she experienced the family's and community's efforts to control and exact perfection from her. At times I felt the urge to exact control from her as well. These all represented, I believe, feelings induced in me, that in turn enabled me to feel, as if from within, the intense, unabating object-relations conflicts in her own family and church—

and in turn to appreciate her actual strides in differentiation against
the cultural grain.

Sessions 9 and 10 were a turning point in her therapy. She
began—as she often did—by talking about discipline problems
with her son. "I'm not getting any better. I've been having bouts of
temper, no control." She had taken the switch to her son, and felt
remorseful: "I was so angry. He doesn't listen. I don't like myself for
losing control . . ." Gradually, we changed the focus from the mis-
deeds of others in her family to how she was feeling. Whereas, in
earlier sessions, she had spent much time displacing and projecting
many of her own problems (control, independence, etc.) onto others, and would only begrudgingly examine these as inner issues, by
the ninth session she needed to devote less time to reviling others:
"I've been really feeling down. My physical therapy is doing no
good. I'm being honest; you asked me how I was doing. I'd like to
use my hand a little bit. I'm walking pretty good, though. My
therapy has come to a standstill. I put in the time and effort, but no
results. It's hard to do more, hard to accept [tearfully] that my hand
might not get better than it is now."

I then talked about the uncertainty everyone (patients and practitioners alike) involved in *any* treatment feels, i.e., the *hope* that
therapy is directly related to continued further improvement, but
likewise the fact that her physical therapist, family physician, orthopedist, rehabilitation doctors, etc., could not *promise* further improvement. I acknowledged the difficulty in accepting the unknown limits of physical therapy. We also talked of the continually
magically tinged expectations from her family and her church community (where the language and anticipated reality of "miracles" to
remedy life's problems are everyday occurrences) for a complete
cure. She wept: "Bicycle . . . I'm supposed to do the bicycle and
some handwriting exercises. The physical therapist didn't make
another appointment for me. It's like she's giving up on me." Carol
experienced the lack of a return appointment as a punishment for
not more fully recovering. I said that I noticed that she was keenly
attuned to the passage of time; several months prior to this session,
she had brought up the imminence of the eighteen-month mark
from the date of her accident—a date that the physicians and
physical therapists said roughly represents the extent of expected
recovery of function.

> It's already the nineteenth or twentieth month since the accident, and I
> feel discouraged. It's like I want to wake up from a big bad dream and

hear somebody say: "It's over now, I can walk right and have the full use of my hand back." But it doesn't happen. After almost two years, I've tried, but I never fully recover from my handicap. At one of my last physical therapy sessions, I asked the therapist: "Is there anything surgical for my hand?" I talked with my husband, too, to see if he had any thoughts about my having surgery for my hand. Not that it would make it perfect, but I might have more use out of it. He said surgery is ridiculous. But I feel I ought to explore everything, not automatically dismiss it. I talked with Dr. V [her local family physician], and he suggested that I wait a while and see whether the physical therapy might improve the arm more. Meanwhile I also talked with the physical therapist. She recommended a local orthopedist, and said she'd talk with him about me if I'd like.

I felt as if she were now asking for my opinion, to be registered in the column of "for" or "against." I said I thought she should discuss the medical issues with Dr. V before taking any action. I also said that I would be willing to continue these therapy sessions irrespective of her decision. I also said that I felt that she was in an especially vulnerable time when she might be tempted to try to find some magical solution to her handicap, and that I felt it important for her to keep this temptation in mind as she was making her decision. She added, almost as a confession: "It's hard for me to accept limits. I don't like to take no for an answer." I reflected that this was very much the same attitude she disliked in her son (and to a degree, in her husband and daughter as well). She was still slowly, and grudgingly, coming to realize that she struggled with her family to try to control the "stubborn" parts of herself.

Near the end of session 10 (two months after session 9), she said with an almost proud smile: "Kids are terrible! Then too, everybody gave up on me [sadly]. I've given up on myself. I gave up on going to the orthopedist. The third of January will be two years since I had the surgery [slip], I mean, since I had the accident. I have better use of my hand, but maybe it won't get better . . ." Her slip revealed the wish to have surgery. She continued, shortly thereafter: "It is hard to give up wishing my hand were perfect. . . . In a recent dream, my hand was perfectly normal. It was a marvelous feeling. But then I woke up, and it wasn't normal. I cried and cried. Crying washes things out. It was good to cry." This was the first time she had been able to *grieve* over her loss of perfection in her hand. We talked about the pain of the mourning process, about the avoidance of that pain by trying to control others for what she can no longer do, and about her wish to regain complete control over herself. We also talked about her feelings of *aloneness* in her grief; that it was as difficult for her family and community to acknowledge the loss (and therefore that she/they had anything to grieve about) as it was for her to grieve for her own irreversible losses.

In session 12, our final meeting, she said wistfully: "It's been two years since the car wreck. It's still hard to accept that my hand won't be all back to normal. I still have that dream that my hand is perfect. It makes me mad that I can't change things. [Earnestly said, then she became sad]. But, I guess I'll have to accept what is, but it's hard." I acknowledged the difficulty of mourning, adding that it would be normal for her perhaps to always have the wish that things could be different, even for her dream to continue for some time. This would not be a sign that she was "crazy," only that it was a powerful wish she would have to learn to live with too.

METAPSYCHOLOGICAL REFLECTIONS
ON THE CASE

The inability to accept loss and to grieve over it—together with the taboo on thinking, let alone voicing, that the disability might be permanent—was a central theme that not only organized the patient's inner fantasy life but characterized her entire social world. (For an excellent review of the literature on psychosocial aspects of spinal-cord injuries, see Friedman-Campbell and Hart 1984; Tucker 1980; Versluys 1980; Werner-Berland 1980.) In the literature on family coping with illness, the concept of "family discrepancy" refers to differences in styles and rates of adaptation between family members (Shapiro 1986; Moos 1979) in coping with the fact of a chronically ill, disabled, or deceased family member. The case discussed in this chapter suggests that this discrepancy—one frequently expressed in blaming if not stigmatizing behavior and social isolation—can often expand to include family, church, local community, and wider culture (see also Stein 1979), becoming a "community discrepancy" or "societal discrepancy." Moreover, as the case demonstrates, this discrepancy cannot be reduced to "purely" cognitive or perceptual differences or expectations among family and church members: rather, these differences in cognition, perception, and expectation are themselves rooted in (shared) unconscious dynamics that make of the patient and her affliction a safe container or "suitable target for externalization" (Volkan 1976). One must thus begin to conceptualize family, community, and cultural *resistances* of which the identified patient or symptom-bearer serves as the focus (see Sander 1979:105; Stein 1982, 1985a).

Wangh's statement that "another person may be used by the ego for defensive purposes" (1962:453) can and must be expanded from the dyad to families and groups (see, for instance, Stein 1985b for a study of how a daredevil diabetic youth was used for fantasy purposes by his entire community). The nature of these narcissistic object ties can profitably be conceptualized in terms of the dynamics of projective identification, externalization, and self-object representations (see also Adams 1985). Sander's formulation of the relation between the patient's inner representational world and external social reality is especially cogent for the present case:

> For the neurotic, inner conflicts are usually enacted and reenacted through the repetition compulsion. He [or she] unconsciously chooses significant others to make his [or her] external reality painful all over again.
>
> The problem clinically is that so often the patient's inner turmoil is then masked by a difficult external reality albeit of his [or her] unconscious choosing. (1979:122)

In a sense, I tried to "do" individual, family, and community therapy by working primarily (although not exclusively) with an individual family/community member. I concur with Sander that in my work with this patient, improvement came "not via the resolution of a transference neurosis but in the reduction of externalizing defenses that in turn makes the internal conflicts that underlie the neurotic interaction more accessible" (Sander 1979:107).

COUNTERTRANSFERENCE ISSUES

No clinical or ethnographic or historiographic (etc.) account is complete without locating the clinician's or observer's or scholar's place in the subject matter: in this case, both the case proper and this narrative constitute the subject matter. Work with this patient was one of the most emotionally demanding, yet exhilarating, encounters I have had with resident physicians, medical students, colleagues, patients, and their families alike. With Searles (1975), Friedman (1985), and many others, I can confidently say that Carol's therapy was also therapeutic for me.

The period of therapy coincided with the agonizing-to-witness decline of my mother's health and her death, together with my arriving at the age of forty. Moreover, the patient's engulfment as a target of projective identification and externalization in her southern Great Plains Baptist family and community both paralleled and reevoked in me my experience of growing up in a Jewish, East

Coast family and community. (I have elsewhere discussed the dynamics of differentiating a sense of self in one's culture of origin;
see Stein 1980.) My own dread of aging, future potential disability,
and death were all made raw and exposed during Carol's therapy:
what I had not wanted to look at in myself, I had now to confront if I
was to help Carol to work through these aspects in herself, her
family, and her community. My early realization that I experienced
her alternately as a "self-object" and as a receptacle of my projective
identification was my first cue both to my own unfinished business
and to the central organizing dynamics in her self, family, and
community.

Just as, early in therapy, Carol was determined that her son not
become like herself, I was equally determined that she not suffer the
fate of my mother. Unable to rescue my own mother, I had set out
to rescue Carol. Early in therapy, I found myself trying super-
humanly to help her repair her children, her marriage, her vocational options, her self-esteem—and not facing the despair that I
could not allow myself to feel in my own life. When I could allow my
mother to be dying, and to begin to let go of her, I could begin to
recognize that the patient's children and husband and church and
rural community were *symbols* to her (as she was to them) and not
people I needed to feel compelled to help her to "fix." In the face of
her vexatious life and my resistance, the patient was simply courageous; her courage "gave" me courage to persist with her in
therapy.

CONCLUSIONS: EXPANDING AND DEEPENING CONTEXTS

The clinician working with individuals, families, groups, institutions, etc., is faced with a bewildering array of models and dogmas,
each vying with the others for claims to truth, methodological
rightness, allegiance, and worthy ancestry (Freud, Jung, Melanie
Klein, Bateson, Minuchin, Selvini Palazzoli, Bowen, to name but a
very few; see, for instance, Kutash and Wolf 1986). Virtually all of
us in the healing professions are "systems" thinkers (whether we use
that current shibboleth, or others). The more vexing question is
how to know what (all) the system is, how one participates in it, and
how to encompass it emotionally (Stein 1987a). In this chapter I
have argued that to limit for ideological purposes what is to be
included in a system perpetuates the problem, for one inadvertently ends up transposing the patient or family's story into the

comfortable "key" of one's own defenses and/or professional loyalties.

When I work with a patient, a family, a physician, a clinic staff, I bring everything I think I know to the understanding of the case. In addition, however, I try to use free-floating attention to allow the patient, the family interplay, the group dynamics, and my own unconscious associations to foster the telling of the story that hitherto could not be told (Miller 1981; Stein 1985f). When the referring physician in the above case asked me to work with this patient on the problem of her depression following her automobile accident, I did not expect to be spending several hours listening to her talk about her exasperation at her children's misbehavior. Yet I trusted that between her chain of associations and feelings and those prompted in me, the hidden connections would emerge.

Watzlawick, Beavin, and Jackson (1967) write that "a phenomenon remains unexplainable as long as the range of observation is not wide enough to include the context in which the phenomenon occurs" (1967: 20–21). While this is certainly true in the above case, I would want to qualify it by insisting that such contexts are not only composed of personal, family, community, and health-care-system units, but rather that these contexts and their various units are themselves *unconsciously linked.* The patient's dream of the mended hand was not her dream alone. It was insuperably difficult for her to mourn her loss because it was so difficult for those in her personal environment to be able to acknowledge that loss, as she represented a part of themselves to them. Their internal factors externalized upon her, compounded those of her own—becoming her own. The unfolding of "the case" illustrates how the linkage between persons, families, communities, and cultures takes place and is continuously reaffirmed. That unfolding gave us profound insight into the social scope of that case—while that selfsame network of cultural relationships and meanings insisted that she, her spine, her will, and her faith were the case alone.

REFERENCES

Adams, B. 1985. Reflections on the external system and/or the internal system or psychoanalysis vis-à-vis family systems theory. *Voices* 21(2):43–51.

Bowen, M. 1978. *Family therapy in clinical practice.* New York: Jason Aronson.

deMause, L. 1974. The evolution of childhood. In *The history of childhood*, edited by L. deMause, 1–73. New York: Psychohistory Press.

Devereux, G. 1969. *Reality and dream: Psychotherapy of a Plains Indian.* New York: New York University Press (orig. 1951).

————. 1978. The works of George Devereux. In *The making of psychological anthropology*, edited by G. Spindler, 364–406. Berkeley and Los Angeles: University of California Press.

————. 1980. *Basic problems of ethno-psychiatry*, translated by B. M. Gulati and G. Devereux. Chicago: University of Chicago Press.

Dundes, A. 1985. The American game of "smear the queer" and the homosexual component of male competitive sport and warfare. *The Journal of Psychoanalytic Anthropology* 8(3):115–29.

Friedman, M. 1985. *The healing dialogue in psychotherapy*. New York: Jason Aronson.

Friedman-Campbell, M., and C. A. Hart. 1984. Theoretical strategies and nursing interventions to promote psychosocial adaptation to spinal cord injuries and disability. *Journal of Neurosurgical Nursing* 16(6):335–42.

Kohut, H. 1971. *The analysis of the self*. New York: International Universities Press.

Kroeber, A. L. 1930. Culture area. In *Encyclopaedia of the social sciences*, vol. 2, edited by E. R. Seligman and A. Johnson, 646–47. New York: Macmillan.

Kutash, I. L., and A. Wolf, eds. 1986. *Psychotherapist's casebook: Theory and technique in the practice of modern therapies*. San Francisco, Calif.: Jossey-Bass.

La Barre, W. 1972. *The ghost dance: The origins of religion*. New York: Dell.

McHolland, J. 1985. Family-systems therapy with an individual. *Voices* 21(2): 61–70.

Mahler, M., and M. Furer. 1968. *On human symbiosis and the vicissitudes of individuation*, vol. 1, *Infantile Psychosis*. New York: International Universities Press.

Miller, A. 1981. *The drama of the gifted child: How narcissistic parents form and deform the emotional lives of their talented children*, translated by R. Ward. New York: Basic Books (orig. 1979).

Moos, R. H. 1979. Evaluating family and work settings. In *Toward a new definition of health*, edited by P. Ahjmed and G. Coelho, 337–60. New York: Plenum.

Sander, F. M. 1979. *Individual and family therapy: Toward an integration*. New York: Jason Aronson.

Searles, H. F. 1975. The patient as therapist to his analyst. In *Tactics and techniques in psychoanalytic therapy*, vol. 2, *Countertransference*, edited by P. L. Giovacchini, 95–151. New York: Jason Aronson.

Shapiro, J. 1986. Assessment of family coping with illness. *Psychosomatics* 27(4):262–64, 269, 271.

Stein, H. F. 1979. Rehabilitation and chronic illness in American culture: The cultural psychodynamics of a medical and social problem. *Journal of Psychological Anthropology* 2(2):153–76.

————. 1980. Bowen "Family systems theory"—The problem of cultural persistence, and the differentiation of self in one's culture. *The Family* 8(1):3–12.

————. 1982. Ethanol and its discontents: Paradoxes of inebriation and sobriety in American culture. *Journal of Psychoanalytic Anthropology* 5(4):355–77.

————. 1985a. Alcoholism as metaphor in American culture: Ritual desecration as social integration. *Ethos* 13(3):195–235.

————. 1985b. The contest for control: A case of diabetes mellitus in multiple contexts. In his *The psychodynamics of medical practice: Unconscious factors in patient care*, 113–42. Berkeley and Los Angeles: University of California Press.

————. 1985c. *The psychoanthropology of American culture*. New York: Psychohistory Press.

————. 1985d. Therapist and family values in cultural context. *Counseling and Values* 30(1):35–46.

————. 1985e. Values and family therapy. In *Families and other systems: The macrosystemic context of family therapy*, edited by J. Schwartzman, 201–43. New York: Guilford Press.

————. 1985f. What is therapeutic in clinical relationships? *Family Medicine* 17(5):188–94.

————. 1987a. Encompassing systems: Implications for citizen diplomacy. *Journal of Humanistic Psychology* 27(3):364–84.

————. 1987b. Farmer and cowboy: The duality of the Midwestern male ethos—A study in ethnicity, regionalism, and national identity. In H. F. Stein and M. Apprey, *From metaphor to meaning: Papers in psychoanalytic anthropology*, vol. 2 of the Series in Medicine, Ethnicity, and Psychoanalysis, 178–227. Charlottesville: University Press of Virginia.

Tucker, S. J. 1980. The psychology of spinal cord injury: Patient-staff intervention. *Rehabilitation Literature* 41(4/5):114–21, 160.

Versluys, H. P. 1980. Physical rehabilitation and family dynamics. *Rehabilitation Literature* 41(3/4):58–66.

Volkan, V. D. 1976. *Primitive internalized object-relations*. New York: International Universities Press.

————. 1981. *Linking objects and linking phenomena: A study of the forms, symptoms, metapsychology, and therapy of complicated mourning*. New York: International Universities Press.

Wangh, M. 1962. The evocation of a proxy: A psychological maneuver, its use as a defense, its purposes and genesis. *Psychoanalytic study of the child* 17:451–69.

Watzlawick, P., J. Beavin, and D. Jackson. 1967. *Pragmatics of Human Communication*. New York: Norton.

Werner-Berland, J. A., ed. 1980. *Grief responses to long-term illness and disability*. Reston, Virginia: Reston Publishing Co.

CHAPTER 3

Witchcraft as a Source of Psychic Trauma: The Intrapsychic Story and Metapsychological Profile of a Ten-Year-Old Victim

MARY MARGARET KELLY AND MAURICE APPREY

INTRODUCTION

Psychotherapists and physicians often hear about witches from their child patients; children's play is fertile ground for conscious and unconscious fantasies about them. And the nonclinician is often fascinated and repelled by any thought of the real existence of witchcraft, which evokes vigorous denial but at the same time a certain unacknowledged dread. The case offered here provides an excellent opportunity to study the reality of sadism and murder in the real world of witchcraft as revealed in the fantasy stories of one of its child victims.

This report is given by the clinical psychologist who treated the traumatized girl and by her supervisor. The former is an American of Irish Catholic descent, the latter a West African child analyst. The therapist grew up in a world honoring technology and reason; the supervisor in a world in which technology and magical beliefs coexist. We agree that at some point in our careers as psychotherapists we must examine what our backgrounds enable us to bring into the work of therapy. Does one's background permit the practitioner to handle therapeutic regression with relative ease? Does the therapist have only his or her own training analyst to rely on to handle regressive situations? A training analysis or psychotherapy is clearly an asset for a therapist to have had; but so, we feel, is a history of having lived in a culture genuinely aware of the power of magic and mystical beliefs.

The effect of one's orientation in this regard became evident at a meeting of a group of physicians, psychologists, and social workers constituting a study group, before whom this case of Blanche was presented. Refreshments had been brought to the meeting, and the presenter mentioned in passing that the child in the case study under consideration had volunteered to bring some ice into the room. Most of those present had never distinguished this child from the many who came and went past the door, but, once identified, she had a surprising effect on members of the group. One refused to touch under any circumstances the drink he was offered, and another could not rest, but kept asking questions and expressing her incredulity about the existence of witchcraft. Another relived her own family situation, having a highly emotional response to the fact that the child under study had been chosen to inherit leadership in the witch coven of her mother. As human individuals, the group members were all stunned. Such things (witchcraft) should not be! Nor should those who practice it escape punishment, as had this child's mother. Magic is understandably incompatible with the world of reason to which the training of most therapists is limited, so it is painful for them to accept the diabolical consequences of witchcraft, although as they appear in a child victim they must be considered.

PART A
Prefatory Note on Magic and the World of Reason

One of the most rewarding aspects of the practice of psychotherapy is also one of its greatest challenges. Inherent in the psychotherapist's work is an ongoing responsibility to question, reexamine, and continually develop aspects of oneself, as well as one's view of the world. Much has been written of the importance to therapeutic relationships of the clinician's self-awareness and sensitivity to the impact of unique aspects of his or her own development. This chapter examines the clinician's response to case material that sharply challenges the fundamental assumptions upon which his or her worldview is based. It describes the challenge to the rational, analytic world of the psychotherapist posed by a nine-year-old psychiatric patient reared in a world of magic, witchcraft, and primitive fantasies and instincts.

The central question concerns the effectiveness of the world of reason (the cultural legacy of the therapist) to defend against the risks and anxieties involved in dealing with the world of magic. This question has implications for our understanding of the cultural context of psychotherapy; the role in the therapeutic dyad of therapist's and patient's cultural legacies; and the consequences of the therapist's identity as a representative of a culture dominated by reason and technology.

Cultural perspectives on reality can be dichotomized into two contrasting worldviews: the primal, animistic world of magic with its concentration on immediate, open, and direct experience of instinct versus the rational world of technology with its emphasis on reason, logic, and renunciation of instinct. Each of these opposing perspectives consists of relentless, enduring, and often unconsciously transmitted rules for optimal adaptation; they offer highly divergent views of reality, with little compatibility between the two in regard to cultural values and norms.

Each frame of reference has its own definition of what is involved in being effective, practical, and down-to-earth. In the world of magic, the most practical approach is an ongoing openness to the beastly realities of primitive life. The technical world offers the practices of denial, devaluation, and repression to buffer direct experience of disturbing animalistic aspects of reality. The practical citizen of the technological world tends toward emotional neutrality, impartiality, and objectivity. To see things clearly in one world is to process primitive emotional stimulation directly; in the other world it is the dispassionate observer who is the clear thinker. The therapist acts as an advocate of the world of reason because his or her goal is to advance the patients' successful adaptation to its realities and demands.

Therefore, our discussion necessitates investigation of how those at home in technology and accustomed to the renunciation of instinct can negotiate case material that, according to their view of the world, is unreal and hence unworthy of attention, something to be minimized and disparaged. Yet the reality of this primal, magical material is so powerfully and relentlessly stimulating and disturbing that these experts must somehow accommodate to the realities of the primitive world. The following case description also raises questions about the effect of these two contrasting perspectives on one's understanding of the patient.

CASE HISTORY

Blanche was nine when admitted to this inpatient psychiatric facility. She presented as a very attractive blonde, blue-eyed, fair-skinned youngster of height and weight average for her age. Her general demeanor was quiet and guarded with peers and adult staff members.

She had been referred for hospitalization for a complete psychiatric review by the community mental health center where she had been in treatment for fourteen months, and to which she had originally been referred, along with her younger sister, Lucinda, to be prepared for a preliminary court hearing charging their biological mother and her boyfriend with sexual abuse. An abuse investigation had been initiated because of Lucinda's unusual sexual behavior in kindergarten, where she had drawn explicit sexual pictures and exposed herself.

The hearing, which took place after about two months of outpatient therapy for both girls, did not result in any charges being pressed against Mrs. W and her boyfriend, Mr. D, as neither girl was able to give testimony to the court. Despite efforts to prepare the girls for the hearing, they could not testify in the presence of their mother. They had to be coaxed into the courtroom, and Blanche covered her eyes with her hands and cried throughout the questioning. The mother continued to deny that any abuse had occurred. No questioning was attempted with Blanche's sister Lucinda, who was then five. Blanche was seven.

Blanche and Lucinda had been placed together in foster care (the family of Mr. and Mrs. R) by the local department of social services when abuse was first reported, and they stayed in foster care with the R's after the preliminary court hearing, in spite of the fact that no official charges were filed; the social service department was concerned about the biological mother's ability to care for them. This concern arose from the extent of sexual abuse the girls reported to their therapist and their foster mother, to whom they began "leaking" information when taken from their biological mother's home. This information concerned rituals that they said took place in their mother's house and involved abuse, mutilation, and ritualistic killing of animals and children, including the murder of an infant sister.

These rituals resembled satanic worship; Blanche described robes, candles, and a noose hanging from the ceiling to warn the children not to talk about what they had seen. There had been drinking of the blood and consumption of body parts (heart and liver) of the dead, according to the children's account. Some corroboration of these events was seen in Lucinda's behavior shortly after she went to live with the foster parents; she became "hysterical," Mrs. R reported, when Blanche cut her finger, screaming that Blanche was not to put the blood on her. Neither girl would eat meat at first, and they still continued not to eat chicken off the bone because of its resemblance to body parts. According to Mrs. R, Lucinda had phobic reactions to books, saying that certain words and numbers could harm her. At times, Lucinda would chant in syllables that resembled Latin. Much of Blanche's play involved themes of the devil.

In videotaped testimony each girl was able to describe in detail to homicide detectives the condition and the site of disposal of the body of a recent victim of a ritualistic killing in their biological mother's home. And in a videotaped interview Blanche reported helping mutilate and kill animals and children. She reported being required to be aggressive toward her sister, who, police investigators felt, was destined to be the cult's next victim. (Videotaped testimony is not admissible evidence in the jurisdiction in which the girls live.)

Police investigation at the time of the children's removal from the home yielded evidence such as bloodstains in the wood of the house and black candle drippings arranged in a circle with an arrow pointing north. Police also found a circle with a six-pointed star prominently displayed on the wall.

Blanche and Lucinda remained in the R's foster family while the department of social services prepared a case for a second court hearing. As evidence against the girls' mother accumulated, the department decided to ask the court for termination of Mrs. W's parental rights.

Blanche and Lucinda seemed quite content in the R's home, and often used the R's last name as their own. At the time of the placement, Mr. and Mrs. R were both in their mid-thirties, with full-time careers; they presented as very warm, nurturing, and concerned individuals. They are both very religious, and Christian (Protestant) values play an important role in their lives. They have one biological son, Harvey, six months older than Blanche, who is described as a well-meaning boy who nevertheless makes a pest out of himself at times. He felt quite competitive with Blanche, and at times would try to irritate and antagonize her, e.g., dropping worms and bugs in her lap and criticizing her ineptitude in certain games and academic activities. At the time of the placement, the R's also had a sixteen-year-old foster daughter, Susan, living with them, but soon after Blanche went to the hospital Susan was expelled from the R's home for running away at night and having sexual relations with her boyfriend.

Blanche made the adjustment to a new school in the R's school district fairly easily. She had problems learning despite average cognitive ability, and was put in a class for slow learners. She presented no behavior problems at school, which had been the case with her school adjustment before she was taken from her biological mother. She was reported to be somewhat shy, and made few friends. In contrast, Lucinda continued the regressed behavior in school that she had engaged in before being taken from her biological mother.

Blanche was greatly relieved when the courtroom procedures ended, but she became even more guarded about discussing painful past experiences. In her twice-weekly outpatient therapy sessions she was extremely reluctant to reflect on her behavior, or to allow the therapist to make interpretations. When the therapist brought up issues either directly or by reflecting on her doll play, Blanche would either put her head down and fall silent or try to divert the therapist's attention. Her doll play in therapy typically revolved around a baby or youngster who was threatened by an evil maternal figure, and whom the therapist was supposed to save, although never actually allowed to do so. Interpretation as to the content or feelings in the play did not seem to help Blanche with her anxiety or to encourage her to reveal more.

The foster mother, the social services worker, and the outpatient therapist agreed that Blanche was a different child at home than she was in school, where she was described as compliant and somewhat inhibited and timid. Her behavioral problems centered in the home; Mrs. R said that Blanche had hit Harvey with a bat and Lucinda with a belt. She also bit Lucinda on the thigh and smashed her hand with a tin can. Blanche also wet her bed three to six times a week. Mr. and Mrs. R responded to Blanche's aggression with time-out procedures that involved putting her in a corner, but they felt this had no effect on her. After ten months in the foster home, Blanche was given medication to modify this aggressiveness (Thiodidazine [Mellaril] 25 mg., three times daily). This was administered to Blanche until she went to the hospital.

The events that precipitated her referral for hospitalization were based on the report of Harvey, her foster brother, that she had engaged in oral sex with the family dog, and that she and her sister had been engaging nightly in oral-genital stimulation. Blanche had threatened to kill Harvey with a kitchen knife if he told his parents about these activities.

At the time of the referral for hospitalization the outpatient therapist expressed the opinion that Blanche's play indicated that she identified with the aggressor and had internalized a "negative, devil image" of herself. In therapy Blanche expressed some ambivalence about her biological mother. Although she spoke of wanting to go back to live with her mother, she also expressed fear at the prospect of doing so. While Blanche appeared to struggle with guilt about the killings in which she had been made to participate with her mother, her therapist reported little sign of remorse associated with her aggression against her sister and her foster brother.

HISTORY OF THE BIOLOGICAL FAMILY

Information regarding Blanche's biological family and her early development is scanty due to limited contact between Mrs. W and personnel from the various community agencies involved in the case. When Mrs. W and Mr. D learned that serious charges were being brought against them they dropped out of sight, but Mrs. W continued to make infrequent phone contacts with the social services worker to inquire briefly about her daughters, and to taunt the worker with her escape from criminal charges.

The limited information available about Blanche and her family is as follows:

Mr. and Mrs. W met as teenage runaways. They were involved with one another for three years before marrying. Blanche was born the year after their marriage. Mrs. W's pregnancy with Blanche was full-term, and delivery was normal. Mrs. W reported being physically abused by Mr. W while pregnant with Blanche, including being kicked in the stomach. Apparently the pregnancy was further complicated by Mrs. W's extreme obesity.

Blanche weighed eight pounds and five ounces at birth, and was described by Mrs. W as a healthy baby who had few childhood illnesses. According to Mrs. W, she walked by twelve months, said "Mama" and "Daddy" at seven months, and was potty-trained at two years of age except for continued nocturnal enuresis.

Lucinda was born two years after Blanche. Mr. W denied paternity despite a reportedly striking resemblance between him and the baby.

Mr. W was reported to have continued abusing Mrs. W and to have deserted the family around the time of Lucinda's birth, when Blanche was about two. Despite physical abuse in the family from the beginning, evidenced satanic cult involvement appeared only after Mr. W left home. It is noteworthy that at age five Blanche had reported being sexually abused by her mother and her mother's boyfriends, graphically describing acts of sodomy. However, the social worker at an inner-city halfway house, to whom Blanche made this complaint, interpreted the report as pure fantasy activated by Blanche's jealousy of her mother because of the attentiveness of her boyfriends.

Little is known of Mr. W's background other than the fact that he was reared in an orphanage. Satanic cult activity can be traced in Mrs. W's family as far back as her maternal great-grandmother.

Mrs. W became a prostitute when she was thirteen years old, and became known as a girl willing to engage in literally any sexual activity for money. Little by little she also gained the reputation of being dangerous and violent. As a teenager, she was placed in a foster home. The circumstances of this placement are unknown. There was a report, however, that on one occasion when she was being driven to her mother's home for a visit, she expressed marked reluctance to enter it. Her mother's home was described as strange, with altars and a black-veiled cross.

Blanche's arrival at the hospital was met with a variety of responses from the clinicians assigned to her treatment team. Reactions ranged from sheer incredulity and denial to voyeurism. The admitting psychiatrist, a faculty member of a major medical center in the city, forbade the exchange of historical information about the case among the clinical staff at the hospital. His rationale was that the case was so dramatic that information would be leaked out of the hospital and eventually find its way to members of the cult within the city, who would then come to do harm to Blanche in the hospital. Even treatment-team members were denied access to Blanche's medical record. A warning not to read the chart was typed and placed on the front cover of her medical record, which was then placed in a secret, locked location in the medical records department. Access to Blanche's chart was granted to the physician, who designated certain nonphysicians who could safely see it. However, throughout Blanche's year-long stay in the hospital, most members of her treatment team never saw her record; this included the art and music therapists, the occupational therapist, the teacher, and the group therapist. Her individual therapist and her primary nurse were granted access to the chart by the physician, who authenticated their privileged status by written authorization filed in the record itself.

The individual therapist at the hospital was extremely circumspect in her handling of the case, steadfast in the belief that the excitement stirred up by reports of the child's history was more a function of the overactive imagination of clinicians involved in the case than of real, verifiable facts. Accordingly, the therapist decided against becoming engrossed in the tantalizing and sensational aspects of the case such as meeting with the homicide detective investigating it or viewing videotapes of Blanche and Lucinda describing the satanic cult activities in which they had participated. She decided not to ask the foster mother and social service worker to repeat the lengthy, fantastic story of the children's lives in the cult. In view of the tendency of many people to exaggerate dramatic aspects of the children's histories, the therapist decided on an unprejudiced encounter with Blanche, without getting involved in minute details of her history. She also declined invitations to present the case, which came from many corners of the professional community.

In contrast, the outpatient therapist involved herself more thoroughly in the case, studying books on witchcraft, including the Satanic Bible, and continuing regular visits with Blanche in the hospital. She gave birth to a baby after Blanche's admission to the hospital, and took her baby there for Blanche to see.

In addition to the therapists and other professionals involved in the treatment of Blanche and her sister, a therapist, Mr. B, had previously been assigned to work with the girls' mother. This referral for counseling was initiated by the school system to help Mrs. W deal with Lucinda's behavior problems. Parent counseling with Mr. B had been going on for several months before Mrs. W's satanic activities were uncovered by local authorities. Mr. B reacted to the abuse charges against Mrs. W with bitter indignation. He insisted that any misbehavior that may have occurred in Mrs. W's house was a product of the girls' misguided attempts to express unwarranted anger and frustration at their mother. At the court session in which Blanche unsuccessfully tried to testify about the many criminal acts that had taken place in her home, Mr. B interpreted her tears and panic on the witness stand as belated shame over betraying her mother. Blanche and Lucinda were age seven and five respectively at the time of their supposed collusion in trying to destroy their mother's good name.

Mr. B's reaction to the girls' reports echoed the account of the social worker given above, who, two years earlier, had been approached by Blanche with a request for help. As previously discussed, she interpreted Blanche's reports of being sexually abused by her mother as being merely a fantasy activated by the girl's jealousy of the attention paid her mother by her boyfriends.

The social worker from the department of social services, Mrs. X, who assumed custody of the girls after they were taken from their mother, was considered a steady cornerstone of composure and support in coordinating the efforts of the many professionals in the case, including police officials, attorneys, and mental health clinicians. Her perspective on her own management of the anguish elicited by the case reveals many facets of her own adjustment. Initially, she had felt disbelief that the girls' mother, who presented as kind, caring, and innocent, could be involved in such atrocities, but this initial stage of unreality was abruptly interrupted by the inexorable flow of unequivocal evidence of evildoing.

The circumstances of the case were often overwhelming, and then Mrs. X would turn to other workers at her agency, asking them simply to listen to how the case was unfolding. However, despite good working relations within the department, the other workers could absorb so little of the story that they were unable to offer adequate support, so she sought support from her family and comfort from her own religious beliefs to enable her to keep on with the case.

While the case was developing most rapidly, all of the professionals involved joined together for several group meetings devoted to free exchange of information and plans for the management of the case. Two distinct features of these meetings appeared as the sessions continued: (*a*) the sharing of religious beliefs; and (*b*) the use of humor—even black humor—to help members adjust to the case material. These helped to maintain the participants' performance, to foster a cohesive working group despite the gruesome nature of the case and despite the wide range of agencies represented in the group membership.

TREATMENT

The following is a description of Blanche's play-therapy work over the course of a one-year hospital stay during which she was seen in therapy three times each week. Briefly, play therapy is a process designed to assist children in telling the story of aspects of their lives that are troublesome to them and over which they have no sense of mastery. Through their play they can repeatedly face and deal with problems. In the course of these playful repetitions for mastery, and in concert with the therapist, new, more adaptive solutions can be achieved. In exploring the sequence of her sessions the authors note that a cyclic pattern emerges in which Blanche repeatedly attempts to directly face the traumas of her past, and to achieve some sense of mastery over them. In the progression of her work there is movement from the use of primitive to mature structures in dealing with the catastrophes of her life, a distinct movement away from an initial protective posture of not knowing, not seeing, not talking, and not trusting. Her final stance was one of relative comfort with awareness and trust.

Blanche's initial refusal to know and see implies anxiety that she might not have enough internal control and support to deal directly with the horrible legacy of her upbringing. Her posture at the end of her hospital stay, indicative of increased ease with self-awareness, reflected increasing stability of internal structures that would make it possible for her to deal with the traumatic material in the sessions. The therapist served in this process as an auxiliary agency promoting the growth of structures that would support accurate seeing and knowing. Most importantly for Blanche, in the final months of treatment, she repeatedly demonstrated creative insight in ways that suggest she was beginning to be able to generalize from one specific learning experience to other spheres of life. For example, in applying knowledge gained in therapy to other aspects of life, she demonstrated the acquisition of stable forms of knowing and profiting from knowing.

Blanche's initial inpatient therapy sessions resembled her previous outpatient work in their guardedness. She was critical of the toys in the playroom, calling them "dumb." She made repeated attempts to avoid going to therapy sessions, and during her walks to the playroom with her therapist, she protested that she did not want to go to therapy. But she always complied, albeit halfheartedly. Once in the playroom, she would scan the room and superficially explore some of the toys, but in less than five minutes she would ask to leave, protesting that the sessions were too boring to be endured. Her mood was generally irritable, and her view of the therapist was one of disdain. This initial phase of disdainful resignation to the requirements of therapy lasted about six weeks.

Her initial reluctance was followed by some doctor play in which the therapist's vision was tested in a series of challenging tests developed by Blanche. These examinations were accompanied by Blanche's self-examination, including blood pressure studies; giving injections to herself; and listening to herself with the toy stethoscope. She also began having to go to the bathroom during each session. Since she was very much afraid of bathrooms, the therapist was asked to "stand guard" while Blanche used the bathroom. These and similar activities designed to evaluate the adequacy of the therapist as well as Blanche's own strength, coupled with the invitation to the therapist to stand guard while Blanche entered places that greatly frightened her, seemed to constitute a transitional phase that focused primarily on establishing sufficient trust to begin to build a working alliance.

This transitional stage was characterized by marked ambivalence about the therapist's seeing Blanche's play. She often asked the therapist not to look at what she was doing, and these requests became a pattern of hide-and-seek that persisted throughout the entire course of treatment. Blanche would hide dolls in various places in the room, and order the therapist to find them. At the start of this hiding game she would gleefully "trick" the therapist by misleading her in the search for the dolls, but gradually she began to demonstrate equal pleasure from giving the therapist accurate clues about their location. Thus, it was only at a very slow pace that Blanche was able to tolerate the therapist's seeing and knowing about hidden things. Very cautiously a pact gradually evolved between Blanche and her therapist, the terms of which involved Blanche's willingness to help the therapist know where to look to discover secret and hidden things. The most salient of the therapist's contributions to this therapeutic pact were patience and absolute consistency.

Several themes were prominent in Blanche's play around the time of the establishment of a tentative working alliance with the therapist. An all-powerful, fantastic young-girl figure, She-Ra, emerged, as did an evil-witch figure and a seemingly endless parade of victims of the evil witch. (There is an idealized children's cartoon character, She-Ra, who resembled Blanche's She-Ra in many respects.) These two figures continued to be central to Blanche's play throughout therapy. Curiously, the witch was without a name during most of the course of therapy, and was referred to by Blanche only as "that lady." She-Ra alternated between being all-powerful and able to defeat the destructive witch, and being overwhelmed by the witch's deadly power. When She-Ra was overwhelmed, she was sometimes rescued by a "helper," and later by a number of helpful figures.

Coinciding with the emergence of the competition between She-Ra and the witch were talks about Blanche's loss of her biological mother. While she was confused about the details of her mother's disappearance, Blanche's understanding was that because of her attempted testimony in court, she caused her mother to be banished forever. She expressed deep guilt about losing her mother, along with loneliness and yearning to have a mother even if it meant returning to her biological mother. The therapist's approach to these disclosures was uncharacteristically direct. Blanche was clearly told that she was not responsible for what happened at her mother's home or for her mother's disappearance.

This candid discussion of Blanche's sense of responsibility for the dissolution of her family was followed by a new form of play that could be described as a jubilant celebration. The dolls all cheered and jumped joyfully about the room, followed by a comment from Blanche that the witch doll had previously scared the dolls, but they were no longer afraid. Despite the initial exhilaration that accompanied the therapist's assertion that Blanche was not at fault for the traumas of the past, the dolls' jubilation was short-lived. They were repeatedly faced with the presence of the malevolent witch in future sessions; but from this point onward, they slowly grew in their ability to see the witch figure for what she was—a dangerous monster. In earlier sessions the witch had easily deceived the dolls about her evil identity. Henceforth, the dolls also became able, at times, to serve a warning function to the idealized She-Ra doll as well as to the baby dolls, who were more easily deceived by the witch doll in Blanche's play.

Beginning in the third month of treatment there was a period of intensified focus on the powerful, benevolent, idealized girl doll, She-Ra. Blanche revealed that she wished she were She-Ra, but could not articulate the motives behind the wish. During several sessions she said that "now is the time for the battle" between She-Ra and the witch figure, but she was unable to stage a battle for many weeks. When the battle finally occurred, it did not actually involve a direct confrontation between the two figures, but instead She-Ra outwitted the witch by stealing her sword and thereby robbing her of her power. She-Ra's life was consequently threatened by the witch; Blanche declared that if She-Ra lost any battles with the witch she would die.

After approximately four months in the hospital Blanche increasingly unconsciously denied her past with the cult, and willfully withheld material about it. In the play, She-Ra continued to be the central figure fighting and killing "bad guys" in the playroom. One peculiar aspect of She-Ra was that she had two distinct personalities: one of the normal, ordinary girl and one of a powerful, idealized, fantasy girl. At times the two personalities were aware of each other, but at other times they were not. She-Ra's clothing and hairstyle were central to her changes in personality; her hair often being loose when she was the fantasy ideal and bound up when she was the ordinary girl. Very rapidly, the other dolls began having changes in identity based on clothing and hairstyle, but their different identities were never as elaborated as She-Ra's.

It was necessary for the dolls to change their identities in order to carry out certain functions such as going to school or attending parties. At times some of the dolls actually exchanged personalities with one another, not deliberately, but while in trances. All of the dolls had periods of dizziness, confusion, and trance states. None were sufficiently clearheaded to be able to understand or articulate what was happening in the playroom, but all went dizzily about the room with no apparent direction to their behavior.

At this point Blanche introduced the farm family into her play. The farm family—a mother, father, son, and daughter—along with their farm animals, repeatedly fell victim to an endless array of traumatic circumstances including car accidents, roller-coaster accidents, mountain-climbing accidents, and towers falling on them. Their only escape from death was being locked up in their farmhouse.

She-Ra eventually came under the influence of the witch several times in therapy. The witch doll would accomplish this transformation by making She-Ra dizzy or making her fall asleep. When She-Ra emerged from her reverie, she had been clothed in the witch's headdress or clothing and had as a result been transformed into an evil doll. Blanche gradually became able to see that She-Ra, though essentially good, did derive some enjoyment from her bad behavior while in trance states induced by the witch.

During this stage there was a reemergence of the importance of secrecy in Blanche's play. For example, She-Ra, as the ordinary girl, was the keeper of a great secret that made her a very important person, and which she shared with no one unless put in a trance by the witch. The secret was her true identity as a girl with superpower. Similarly, there was renewed discomfort with the therapist's seeing the dolls' play, especially when they underwent their changes in identity. Simultaneous with this renewed emphasis on secrecy was an increase in Blanche's nightmares. She awakened nightly, screaming in the midst of obviously horrible nightmares.

At this point in her therapy she produced material indicative of significant sibling rivalry. Sister dolls deceived, tricked, fought, and killed each other. Blanche made continual inquiries about the other children who came into the therapist's office, even asking about future patients who might replace her.

The significance of siblings in this rivalrous play was multi-faceted. At the Oedipal level, sibling dolls killed each other to win primacy with a prestigious male figure. Also, Blanche had only recently learned from her foster parents that she was permanently expelled from their home, and would not be allowed to return there. She learned, too, that the foster family was permitting Lucinda to remain with them. Thus, in her external world she experienced a significant object loss, having been pushed out of the home in favor of her sister. Finally, evidence uncovered by police investigators pointed to the strong likelihood that prior to the girls' removal from their mother, Lucinda was being groomed to become the cult's next sacrificial victim—in a killing Blanche was being primed to carry out.

In the playroom, as threats and hostility continued to be exchanged between sister dolls, Blanche announced that the older sister doll, along with several others, was preparing for a special sinister ceremony at which the younger sister was guest of honor. Although the preparations became increasingly threatening and morbid, when the final ceremony took place it was transformed at the last minute into a wedding ceremony in which the younger sister married the handsome and powerful male doll that both girls had competed for. A past reality became turned around in the play, thus instituting reparation and restitution.

During this phase of play, all of the dolls whirled about the playroom in trancelike states of muddled consciousness. Their will was not their own, and their behavior was not self-directed; instead, a vague force or power had them all under its influence.

Eventually, Blanche herself played at being a ghost. She relished her ghostlike status because it allowed her to become invisible at will. Out of this dizziness emerged a period of reenactments of animal torture and sacrifices and ritualistic murder of children. Blanche repeatedly played out scenes in which dolls were lured into haunted houses from which they never returned. One by one the dolls in the playroom disappeared under a sacrificial table designed by Blanche. Limbs and body parts became separated from the victims. She repeatedly played a game of "now you see it (the baby doll victims), now you don't." Meanwhile, parent dolls incoherently roamed the playroom searching in vain for their lost children.

Blanche warned the therapist about the play, prefacing it with the statement, "I'm gonna scare you." The function of the warning was not to frighten the therapist but to assess her durability; to signal that considerable fortitude would be required in order to lend Blanche the strength to face these horrors. Themes of cannibalism were prominent as well. The dolls were repeatedly placed in a stew pot. Blanche made sinister meals for the remaining dolls and would not let them watch her prepare the food lest they be aware of what it was. A big-sister doll came to the table and ate the food and became ill because it was "the wrong thing to eat." However, the little-sister doll "peeked" during the cooking process and refused to eat the food. Although she did not become ill, she was denied any nourishment by Blanche, the cook. Occasionally the evil doll who had put the other dolls in the pot was trapped in the pot herself.

During this period of Blanche's first exposure of the horrors of her past, she became quite dependent on the therapist, asking for much assistance during the play sessions and having considerable difficulty separating from the therapist after sessions were over. She repeatedly asked the therapist to adopt her and become her new mother. Her fantasies of adoption by the therapist included never again being "scared by a mother." She voiced a fantasy that the therapist would be an indulgent mother who would allow her to do whatever she wished.

This phase of great dependence on the therapist was followed by increasingly intense ambivalence toward her. Although Blanche often refused to leave therapy sessions, she was frequently highly reluctant to begin them. Often when entering the playroom she would make pronouncements regarding how much time she was willing to spend in therapy, e.g., "I want just three minutes of therapy today." Despite her limit-testing around the issue of her time in therapy, she responded positively to firm, gentle reminders of the therapy rules.

At this point in her therapy Blanche started play activities that involved direct competition with her therapist. Initially, when she discovered that she could compete successfully against the therapist, she became elated, and maneuvered the competitive games so that she inevitably won. Only after many weeks of invariably winning all competition with her therapist did Blanche begin to vary the outcome of these games so that both therapist and patient could win.

It was also at this point in therapy that Blanche produced her only unsolicited memory of her biological mother. She asked the therapist to draw a picture of the ocean with the sun setting into it and birds flying over it. Blanche then drew two figures in the water and labeled them her mother and herself as a tiny baby. She described being held in her mother's comforting and powerful arms, but at the same time being terrified by the relentless movement of the ocean tides. She described her mother as holding her gently but firmly until she was no longer frightened by the ocean and could even enjoy the water around them. The image was one of a protective parent lovingly holding her baby but surrounded by danger and unrest. There was an ideal quality to the memory, in that the mother was, on the one hand, empathic to her baby's needs for protection and security but, on the other, exposing her to the natural ups and downs of the external environment at the infant's most comfortable pace. Blanche seemed to be evaluating these same functions as performed by the therapist in the treatment: protecting, and allowing the child to genuinely experience its world. And she seemed to be comparing the therapist's efforts to powerful and ideal internal criteria.

Around the midway point in therapy (after approximately five to six months), Blanche's play became increasingly fragmented. Each session was composed of a series of miniature dramas that would inevitably abruptly end without resolution. As the story line of one drama reached the point of greatest conflict and tension, it was abruptly replaced with a different story line. Once again, the doll characters in the stories lost their own continuity of identities. However, in contrast to the first period of massive confusion among the dolls, this time they were less dizzy and more spontaneous and willful in their behavior. The dolls fought with one another, victimized one another, and became one another, sometimes losing, sometimes exchanging, identities. Many times they lost their identities and lost control over themselves and their behavior when they changed clothes or moved to different locations in the room. They were more easily brought under the complete control of other dolls, but rather than dizzily proceeding with duties imposed by a vague force, they seemed more aware and more invested in their trance duties.

At times during the play Blanche would hold a doll in front of the therapist and directly ask her for the doll's identity. Frequently, the doll's identity was to be a secret from the therapist. In this case, if the doll's true identity was revealed, the doll would fly into a rage, killing other dolls as well as farm animals. At other times, Blanche appeared to have sufficiently dissociated herself from a story fragment she had just played out so that she had apparently no real recollection of the identity of the doll in her hand, even if it had just been the center of her story. At times the dolls would poignantly ask the therapist, "Who is Blanche?"—revealing the presence of clear depersonalization.

Concurrent with this direct questioning of the therapist to identify the dolls in the playroom, there emerged a new central figure, the Little Guard Girl, a small girl doll who had many responsibilities in the playroom. She coached the therapist in answering the questions of other dolls about their true identities. She also knew the dolls' secrets, and was inclined to share them with the therapist. She intervened when the other dolls became aggressive, and also was able to prevent some of the accidents that happened to the victim dolls. For example, the farm family's car was forever going out of control and plunging the family to its death over cliffs and into buildings, but the Little Guard Girl was able to tell the therapist when and where to place her hand to catch the car and its occupants before an accident could occur.

One of the Little Guard Girl's functions had previously been sporadically carried out by a benevolent, trustworthy, but not very powerful father doll. He was occasionally able to save children and animals from danger by taking them far away from dangerous areas to places of safety. But the Little Guard Girl's fate was not so happy; when she divulged the secret identity of some of the dolls, she was beaten to death by the dolls. After her death, most of the other dolls died mysteriously over a period of about a week. Sometimes the dolls would directly announce to the therapist that "Today is the day I am going to die." Some of them were replaced by their spirits or ghosts, who flew around the room, haunted the dollhouse, and frightened the few survivors of the death and destruction in the playroom. The ghosts were capable of luring children and animals into their haunted houses and then killing and eating their victims.

Blanche's mood was one of severe depression (frequent crying, sadness) during this period of therapy. Play figures emerged only to be killed in accidents or to die mysteriously. Blanche destroyed some of her own clay productions made earlier in therapy. She protested violently when the therapist tried to stop the destruction and pick up the broken pieces of clay and put them in a secure place. She renewed her questioning about the therapist's other patients and wept regularly at the prospect of never again having a family or a mother. Her nightly enuresis, which had abated for three months, resumed. During the next month she produced several additional sea drawings of her mother and herself as an infant. The hide-and-seek games that had persisted from the early sessions were now punctuated with whispers, cries, and screams when Blanche hid, waiting for the therapist to find her. She often called out as though she were being tortured, and when asked about this, she denied its significance, saying that she was only pretending to be hurt in order to trick the therapist.

The doll figures in her play were always surrounded by danger. A benign father figure made a few brief appearances to move the easily victimized farm animals and children to safer places. The mother figures pushed their children to their death in haunted houses, and at the same time grieved over their demise. Subsequently, the mother figures themselves died.

An enduring theme during this time was Blanche's assessment of the therapist's ability to help, to be strong enough to look directly at the horrors of her life and powerful enough to help her somehow come to terms with them. Occasionally, the baby dolls asked the therapist to help them be big enough to be unafraid of the danger of their world. Blanche routinely accused the therapist of no longer caring for her because she had begun treatment of another girl on Blanche's ward. She often cried, saying that she had lost her therapist. Clearly she could not tolerate the notion of being an ordinary patient who must share the therapist's attention and concern with another child. She became furious at the therapist, and was inconsolably dejected and irritable in the sessions and on the ward.

For several weeks her play sessions centered on the re-creation of a hopeless, dangerous, violent world impossible to understand or control, and on repeated evaluation of the therapist's ability to see that world clearly. This sequence was followed by one highly unusual session in which Blanche quite uncharacteristically relinquished the toys in favor of talking about her past life. In this session after entering the playroom she asked to see the old, damaged clay pieces she had savaged in an earlier session. She asked about the possibility of repairing them, and talked with the therapist about restoring them some day. She spoke hopefully about the chances of putting the pieces back together successfully, but did not try to do so at that time.

Sitting next to the therapist, she then tried, with stumbling and stuttering words, to talk about her mother. She gave painful accounts of her mother's violence, and then denied what she had said. She tried to draw a picture of painful past events, but could not. She expressed deep regret and shame for her own role in the violence, and then reported feeling that she had caused the loss of two mothers: her biological mother because of her confessions to the police and her foster mother because of her aggression.

This discussion continued with encouragement from the therapist, who indicated understanding of how hard it was for Blanche to remember how things had been in the past and remarked about how much courage it took to do so. She also made therapeutic comments on the confusion Blanche must have experienced when the grown-ups in her family, who were supposed to protect her from frightening things, actually involved her in terrifying activities. It was also emphasized that the grown-ups were in charge at her house, and no matter how important her status may have been, as a child she could not be blamed for what she was made to do, even though she might feel responsible.

Blanche alternately blamed herself and her sister for their mother's disappearance. Had they not spoken up about what was going on in the house, Blanche would not now be locked in a hospital without a mother. The therapist told her directly, as she had previously done, that her testimony was unrelated to her mother's disappearance, that the police had found out independent of her testimony what her mother had done, and that in order to avoid going to jail her mother had fled. For several weeks after this unusual "talk" session, Blanche prefaced each play session with feeble and sometimes pathetic requests for the therapist's help. She began each session asking "Can you help me?" and then rather frantically went about the room identifying various activities that would require the therapist's assistance. As soon as one activity was begun she would find yet another. Then came a play session in which the mother doll left her family after stuffing her children into a large kettle. The children's father rescued them and flew off with them, far away from the mother he had put on a dangerous roller coaster.

For the first time in her eight months of therapy Blanche put the witch's robe on the witch doll; she had previously taken care to avoid any contact with the black and red robe. At the same time she began to wear an old raincoat that hung in the playroom and that she had identified as belonging to her therapist. The witch doll proceeded to put a spell on She-Ra, and while She-Ra was under this spell the tiny farm family became corrupted. Its members began to deceive and trick the witch and She-Ra and then stole their clothes and possessions. Blanche later revealed that the family members were performing these acts under the power of another doll, who had triumphed in the wars of sibling rivalry by killing her sister.

She-Ra soon found out about the little family's deception and retrieved all the stolen goods. The farm-family father then apologized to the witch for the family's deception, but died immediately. He was wrapped in the witch's robe and carried off in a hearse. His daughter fared much better, immediately becoming a powerful queen equal to She-Ra in status. Her elevation allowed her to provide for the remaining family members, who were poor and hungry.

The farm family continued to deceive She-Ra in subsequent sessions by luring her into their house, stealing her possessions, and then giving them to the witch doll. The little farm family was bound to do whatever evil activity (mainly stealing) the witch doll required of them, even if they did not want to do it.

Blanche asked more and more for the therapist's help, and told her how to help the dolls. It was at this time that Blanche had her first hide-and-seek game without horrible screams in approximately two months. Gradually over the next month the screams were replaced by ghosts, and the hide-and-seek game became a hunt for the spirits of lost children. She-Ra was eventually drawn into the search for the spirits.

Blanche pretended to be a ghost herself, delighting in her ghostly status in the hide-and-seek game because it gave her the all-important quality of becoming invisible; in this way she could keep secrets from the therapist. A new twist was added to the games when the Little Guard Girl surfaced briefly to give the therapist magic eyeglasses that would enable her to see Blanche at all times, even when she was "invisible."

Blanche began drawing again, producing for the therapist a "feeling chart," which consisted of a number of faces, each of which depicted a different emotion. Each face was then labeled with its corresponding emotion, and blocked off from the other faces with heavy lines. Blanche told the therapist how she was to respond when Blanche was experiencing each emotion. She taped the chart on the playroom wall, and in subsequent sessions made check marks next to the emotion she was feeling.

At the same time that she created a chart to discriminate among emotions, her play reflected continued confusion about each doll's identity; She-Ra and the witch doll exchanged identities. When asked how She-Ra and the witch were different, Blanche responded that the latter was in control of the personality changes, and that dolls who became like her became evil. She then, after nine months in therapy, named the witch doll: Evil Lady.

Once named, the witch doll gradually lost some of her power. In the session in which she was given a name, she was shot, and was mysteriously struck on the head while in the process of imprisoning She-Ra in her evil tower. Further evidence of erosion of the witch doll's power was seen in the reemergence of the Little Guard Girl, who was able to rescue She-Ra from the witch's prison. Frightening hide-and-seek games persisted, typically occurring in the final minutes of each play session.

Blanche's affect improved considerably at this point in therapy, in contrast to the substantial depression, hopelessness, and occasional extreme anger at the therapist that had characterized the previous three months of work. A new theme was repeated in Blanche's play involving interactions between mother dolls and their children, initially taking the form of interactions between a mother horse and her foal. In the play the mother horse would wear the black and red robe of the witch; this conveyed special status as well as the ability to alter her identity. The mother repeatedly tried to put a similar robe across the back of her foal, who was frightened by it and tried to run away. Blanche's explanation of its fear was that the foal could not do all the things the wearing of the robe required. Specifically, she reported that the foal was unable to make the changes in identity necessary for carrying out the tasks required by the wearing of the robe.

In future sessions the mother animals were often impatient with their babies' discomfort with the special robe. Some baby animals stumbled and collapsed under its weight. The mothers scolded them for being clumsy with the robe, but She-Ra intervened after a short time, explaining to the mothers that their babies were too young to understand the robe and to know what to do with it. The mother replied that the robe was most important because it could protect and sometimes hide the babies. Besides, wearing the robe allowed the baby to become just like the mother. She-Ra explained that the babies were just too young to be like their mothers; She-Ra then proceeded to give the mothers parenting lessons, instructing each "how to be nice to your baby," and simultaneously teaching each baby how to hide and be safe from danger without the robe.

Coinciding with this play was play of a successful escape of a little girl doll from her family. She was aided by the Little Guard Girl in running to a train station and riding a train to find her father, who would keep her safe. The Little Guard Girl stayed behind at the station to thwart the little girl's mother and grandmother, who were pursuing her.

The ninth month of therapy was a time of considerable optimism for Blanche. She spoke hopefully for the first time about her chances of being placed with a new mother. She continued her competitive games with the therapist, varying the outcome of each game. She also continued to request much assistance from the therapist in play activities, and in helping to save dolls from various troubles and threats. She again asked the therapist to become her mother, and was able to listen to the explanation of the special rule that prevents a therapist from ever becoming the mother of a patient.

Instead of becoming her mother, the therapist helped Blanche draw up a list of attributes she wanted her new mother to have. Included was the ability to cook good food; attractiveness; and willingness to let Blanche visit her sister, Lucinda. Blanche also wanted a mother who would keep her forever and never give her up. But most important was the wish for a mother who would not play tricks on her—in other words, one who was clear about good and evil. While drawing up specifications for the mother she wanted, she set about repairing the clay items she had tried to destroy several months earlier, and worked with the therapist's help until they were restored to her satisfaction.

In one session during this stage of play she recalled the mare who had so impatiently insisted that her foal wear the special robe. She reported to the therapist that this horse mother was ashamed of herself. She explained that the mare always hugged her baby, but only knew how to hug it in a "strange" way. The mother was ashamed that she could not hug her baby in a normal fashion. In the same session Blanche anxiously admitted that she missed her biological mother greatly, although she had sometimes frightened and confused her. The conversation focused on how one can feel many different but powerful feelings about the same person. Blanche began to apply this knowledge to her understanding of her feelings of love and resentment toward her sister.

The theme of passing on the trappings of evil power from mother to child persisted. In one session, a little girl was given the Evil Lady's headdress to try on; it gave her the power to fly, but scared all the other dolls away from her. More ghosts emerged in the playroom, and Blanche continued at times to pretend that she was herself a ghost. She began to talk, though always vaguely, about her frightening dreams. The pace of her play sessions quickened and she began volunteering very limited bits of information about her fear of ghosts, not only to her therapist but also in her music and art therapy classes. A condensed version of her fears involved thinking about death and about the spirits of children who had died. She reported that she knew that when a person dies, his spirit leaves his body, and if one stays close to the body, one can feel the power of the dead person's spirit. She also said that under certain circumstances dead people's spirits stay around a given area and haunt its inhabitants. She likened these fears of such haunting ghosts to her nightmares.

At this time the therapist introduced an intervention that consisted of Blanche's joining with the therapist at the end of each session to find a place or object in the room in which they could pretend to place all the frightening ghosts who came to trouble her in her dreams. Blanche readily identified a box in which the play ghosts could reside, a place where they could rest peacefully and feel they belonged, so that they would not come out until she wanted to include them in her play.

The final three months of therapy began with a very brief re-emergence of denial. Blanche indicated that all she had revealed in prior sessions was untrue. This claim was quickly followed by sessions in which several dolls came before the therapist to make graphic reports of mutilation and abuse they had suffered. Blanche would cry out that they were telling lies. These sessions were immediately followed by active work on Blanche's part concerning her guilt for what had happened in the coven. She sometimes referred to herself as a monster, once again going through a period of depression but much less severe than the depression of three months earlier.

In her play she arrested herself and maternal figures in the room. A little girl doll escaped as a contrasting figure in the play and hurt the other dolls again and again. Her misbehavior was not deliberate, however; her evildoing had an almost accidental quality. In fact, Blanche often referred to the little girl's "making another mistake." At times Blanche asked the therapist to intervene and halt the little girl's aggressive acts. The Little Guard Girl surfaced again to occasionally arrest the evil little girl or otherwise stop her. When the Little Guard Girl was in danger, the therapist was asked to protect her; this rescuing function contrasted sharply with Blanche's earlier play, in which the Little Guard Girl perished when she tried to exercise her control functions. Gradually Blanche herself began to assume some of the control functions, occasionally stopping the evil little girl's aggression against the other dolls in the playroom. At the same time Blanche expressed fear that she and her mother would be sent to Hell for what they had done. She revealed that she liked to pretend that Jesus was her father because she had no father of her own.

She became increasingly curious about anger, and expressed fear of the anger of each of the female members of her treatment team as well as of the therapist's. When asked what she thought would happen if any of these people became angry at her, she could not identify any behavior with which they would frighten her, but she nevertheless continued reporting fear of their anger. She was visibly shaken when asked what might happen if the therapist were to become angry with her; although this was simply a reflection of her own question to the therapist, she was shocked that the therapist would even discuss the question. She replied that she had thought that therapists never get angry, and subsequently launched into a series of discussions with the therapist and other trusted staff members about what a youngster typically could expect of adults when they are angry, and how grown-ups in general, and mothers in particular, manage their anger toward children.

Blanche began mothering the baby dolls, feeding and clothing them. She talked about how she would punish her babies when she became a mother, and described very nonpunitive disciplinary techniques such as those used on the ward. She confided in the therapist, though, that they both knew that deep inside her she could become very angry. Nevertheless her doll play remained quite benevolent.

In the closing months of therapy, she began having regular tea parties at the beginning of each play session, indicating that they were given for her by her therapist. She also began putting the frightening ghosts in the teapot at the end of each session rather than using older resting places for them. She told the therapist that if they were in the teapot, the therapist could burn them up on the stove between sessions. With the tea parties came a marked reduction in the previously frantic pace of the sessions; after each one Blanche would look after her dolls. She also staged hide-and-seek games in which she would hide and then pretend that ghosts were hiding in various parts of the playroom. Her nightmares had subsided in frequency as well as intensity, but did occur at least two or three times a week.

During this relatively calm time Blanche learned that the social service worker had finally found her an adoptive family; she was delighted, and though very shy at first during visits with this family, she quickly responded to their warmth and the sense of security and stability they conveyed. In the final weeks of her hospital stay, while the family came to visit and Blanche occasionally went to their home, a new theme was included in the play sessions. One of the young dolls Blanche had been nurturing, one she identified as the Little Guard Girl's sister, began having long-awaited visits from her mother. She and her mother were not allowed to live together and could visit only occasionally. She adored her mother, but the other dolls shared a terrible secret—that the mother was a horrible monster. She-Ra, the ideal girl, warned the daughter, but she would not listen. While the daughter doll was terrified of making her mother angry, she was completely devoted to her.

During this play were two sessions in which Blanche lashed out at the therapist. The verbatim content of her protests was what one might expect her to want to say to her biological mother: she accused the therapist of "bossing" her and telling her to do horrible things. She vigorously insisted that she was tired of being bossed, and tested limits by refusing to leave the room and trying to smash some of the toys. After these outbursts she ran sobbing to the therapist, crying out that she did not mean to say those words but was too angry to hold them back. The therapist told her that she understood that Blanche needed to show her how very disappointing, confusing, and frustrating grown-ups in her life had been, and that she needed to show the therapist how it felt, telling her therapist what she would like to tell those grown-ups. The therapist also indicated that she understood that by trying to ruin her toys Blanche was demonstrating her need to destroy old painful memories. She encouraged the child to share these urges in words rather than in action.

In the meantime, the daughter doll, finally taking in the message of the other dolls that her mother was a monster, resolved her dilemma by reporting to the therapist that the daughter doll would soon be leaving the hospital, but that her mother was "too sick to ever leave the hospital." Blanche told the mother doll not to worry about her daughter because Blanche had taken good care of her in the mother's absence, and she would be all right.

At the same time, She-Ra and some other dolls were playing out a final attempt to master the intense ambivalence about seeing and not seeing. She-Ra made final checks of the haunted areas of the playroom. All of the ghosts had taken up residence under the table.

The dolls were divided into the blind, who, because they could not see were unafraid of facing the haunted place; and the sighted, who were afraid of what they might see there. Neither type of doll could successfully deal with the haunted place; the sighted were too frightened, and the blind could not find their way, but would stumble over obstacles in their path and then become disoriented and lost.

Finally, Blanche invited the therapist to accompany She-Ra in looking directly at the haunted place, which was full of skeletons and man-eating fish. Before doing this, they agreed that they must be able to keep their eyes open and see in order to travel safely, but once they came to the haunted place they must remember that the ghosts within now had a resting place and so could not harm them, regardless of how frightening their appearance might be. She-Ra carefully traveled to the place and courageously entered it, emerging unharmed and victorious because, Blanche explained, She-Ra kept her eyes open and kept remembering that the ghosts were where they belonged.

DISCUSSION

In reviewing the course of Blanche's therapy sessions, it is clear that her work did not progress in a linear fashion from a beginning to an ending point at which she was far more open and effective in dealing with her problems. Instead, her work is best understood as a series of cycles, each of which reflected her central concerns—as clearly as she was able to portray them—as well as reflecting her methods for dealing with those concerns.

Each play cycle began with efforts at patent denial of her traumatic history and its emotional aftermath. This period of denial was followed by evaluation of the therapist's stability, trustworthiness, and endurance. With the therapist's repeatedly renewed status as a reliable anchor in reality, Blanche was able to move to the next point in the cycle, which could be described as a reentry into the world of madness she had inherited from the cult. During this reentry period she worked at exposing the events of the past; in doing so, she also demonstrated coping mechanisms she had used in the past to deal with trauma, and those she was employing in the present. For example, besides revealing the killing of children in her doll play, she depicted the diminished consciousness, depersonalization, and compartmentalization that provided such a barrier of protective obscurity that she was able to survive her trauma.

In spite of her efforts to resolve the madness, she would inevitably reach the limit of her resources, and come to a point in the cycle where she could not marshal the strength to face the increasingly horrifying images she was recalling. Then she would begin the next cycle with a period of denial evoked by the terror of her memories. Thus, in a progression of cycles traumatic material was repetitively reapproached, each cycle bringing increasingly direct depictions of past traumas and their impact on her. As she reviewed them, Blanche was able to explore them from the perspective of both aggressor and victim, and she gradually became able to study in play the relative effectiveness of various coping mechanisms in reducing anxiety and promoting good adaptation.

Reparations, restitution, and reaction formation emerged as prominent themes in Blanche's play. With the completion of each cycle, she showed an expanding openness to the offerings of the new world around her in developing solutions to problems. Her play revealed identifications with the therapist and reduction of identifications with her mother and the cult. The presence of new introjects (inner mental figures) was revealed in the increasingly benign doll figures in later play themes.

The ever-present playful competition with the therapist, and increasing identification with her, suggest the presence of Oedipal negotiations acting as a prelude to superego formation. Blanche appeared to have grown sufficiently to be ready for conscience development. The play revealed Blanche's entry into latency, where there was some capacity for repression of horrible past events, some degree of sublimation potential, and some degree of attachment to same-sex peers. Consistent evidence of each of these accomplishments could be found in Blanche's adjustments during her final months in the hospital.

PART B

TERMINAL DEVELOPMENTAL PROFILE
BLANCHE W—AUGUST 15, 1978

The metapsychological profile, developed by Anna Freud, is a diagnostic technique that can be used for the assessment of developmental psychopathology in children. A terminal developmental profile is generally done following treatment, and integrates data from the therapy with preliminary diagnostic information to obtain as comprehensive and precise an understanding of the child's functioning as possible. The profile covers a wide range of areas of function, including physical and cognitive development, familial and social factors, and internal psychodynamic concerns.

Family Constellation

Father, Mr. W
Date of birth, March 24, 1957

Mother, Mrs. W
Date of birth, January 31, 1959

Sister, Lucinda
Date of birth, May 13, 1980

LIST OF REFERRAL MATERIAL

Outpatient Therapist's Report
Social Services Department Report
School Records

I. PRELIMINARY STATEMENT

Blanche W had just had her ninth birthday when admitted to an inpatient child psychiatric facility in the Washington, D.C., area. Unique aspects of her history center on her birth into a satanic cult that she was expected to lead on becoming an adult, inheriting the dominant position in the coven from her mother, Mrs. W, who had inherited it in her turn from her mother.

Blanche had been required to participate in the cult's activities, which included orgiastic sexual behavior among adults, children, and animals; ritualistic torture, mutilation, and killing of animals and children as sacrifices; and cannibalism. Some of the children sacrificed had been kidnapped; some were offspring of cult members.

This profile focuses on observations of Blanche W during her year in the hospital, with such questions as: What are the likely long-term effects of this extreme and chronic trauma on this youngster's development? To what extent will continued exposure to trauma tamper with the psychic quiescence of latency? How will this young girl negotiate the changes and stresses of puberty's onset? The hospital treatment team had serious concerns about this patient's capacity to adjust to life in a foster family in view of her aberrant family upbringing in the cult.

II. THE REFERRAL

Blanche W was referred to the hospital by her outpatient therapist and the foster parents, Mr. and Mrs. R, with whom she and her sister had lived for fourteen months after being taken from their biological mother. At the time of hospitalization Mr. and Mrs. R expressed reluctance to accept Blanche back into their home, and approximately six weeks later they confirmed to Blanche that they would not take her back.

Doctor G had been seeing Blanche and her sister separately in weekly outpatient therapy sessions since they had been taken from their mother. The initial referral was made to help the girls make the transition from living in a cult to living with a foster family. Lucinda's presenting problem indicated psychosis, with looseness of thought and bizarre behavior, but Blanche's symptoms included aggressive behavior directed at her sister and her foster parents' only biological son, who was her age; she hit him and occasionally fought with Lucinda. She also reportedly threatened to kill Harvey, the son, with a kitchen knife if he disclosed the girls' sexual activities, which included nightly oral-genital stimulation between the girls and oral sex with the family dog. The foster parents saw Blanche as the instigator of these activities and Lucinda as a passive victim.

III. DESCRIPTION OF THE CHILD

Blanche, an attractive blonde, blue-eyed youngster of average height and weight, seemed timid and reticent. She tended to isolate herself on the ward, preferring solitary play to involvement with peers. When others initiated contact, she was polite but extremely quiet. She refused to answer questions about her past by solemnly and slowly shaking her head when questioned.

Blanche was kind to the other children on the ward, freely sharing her toys and being easily victimized by aggressive youngsters. She seemed at a loss for any active ways of dealing with abuse from other children, and never exhibited aggressive behavior toward them, even when confronted by the most annoying and provocative youngsters. She was reserved with authorities, but compliant. When asked to do things she disliked, e.g., bathing, she occasionally became sullen and dilatory.

When pressed to talk about feelings, she verbalized indignation about being put in the hospital. She was particularly resentful toward her outpatient therapist who, she felt, had betrayed her by sending her there. She solemnly assumed responsibility for the fighting in her foster home, and at times shared desperately remorseful and hopeless feelings of having lost her sister and her foster family because of her aggressive behavior while in foster care.

IV. PERSONAL AND SOCIAL HISTORY

Blanche was the first child of Mrs. W, a central figure in a satanic cult based in Vienna, Virginia, a suburb of Washington, D.C. Relatively little is known about Blanche's early childhood because Mrs. W quickly eluded officials, owing to the threat of criminal charges pending against her. It appeared that Blanche had been delivered in good health after an uneventful pregnancy. Mrs. W dated Blanche's first words—"Mama" and "Daddy"—at seven months, and told of her walking by twelve months and achieving daytime bowel and bladder control by the age of two, although she had never managed bladder control at night.

As far as can be determined, Blanche was born into the favored position in the cult, apparently inheriting it as a firstborn daughter from at least four generations. Very little is known about her father, who had apparently met her mother when both were teenagers "hanging out" in a rough part of the city. He remained with his family for two or three years, but left around the time of the birth of the second child, Lucinda. He was described as being physically abusive.

Blanche had been scarcely noticed by school officials, although she was a poor achiever. Her sister's bizarre and explicit sexual behavior was noted early in school, however. After being taken from their mother, both girls apparently adjusted quickly to the foster home, even asking if they could use the R's name as their own. Although Lucinda continued to be loose and disorganized in thinking, tangential and rambling in her speech, and regressed and bizarre in her behavior, the R's felt that she had formed an emotional bond with them; but they experienced Blanche as withdrawn and aloof. They were alarmed by her threat to kill their son, and felt that she was exerting a powerful negative influence over Lucinda. Their fears prompted her referral to the hospital.

V. POSSIBLY SIGNIFICANT ENVIRONMENTAL FACTORS AS TO THE CAUSATION OF THE ILLNESS

1. Since Blanche's father was abusive and had deserted his family when Blanche was only two, violence appears to have imme-

diately assumed a central role in her world. What, therefore, are the chances of this child's being able to establish any sense of basic trust in others?

2.　Blanche and her sister were made to participate in the ritualistic mutilation and killing of animals and children. One might wonder about the chances children with such a background had to develop a normal perspective as to the value of human life, and what the effect would be on the fostering of repressions appropriate for subsequent sublimational potential.

3.　Blanche was described in the cult as a child of Satan who originated "down below." How does such a sense of being rooted in evil affect the development of the superego and the self?

4.　Blanche was born into a position of great status and authority in a culture of violence. With so inflated a sense of importance and value in this subculture, what is the likelihood of her casting aside this world of darkness in favor of membership in a world in which she is an ordinary girl whose status is like any other's?

5.　Investigators interviewing Blanche and her sister quickly realized that they were experienced participants in every possible form of sexual activity involving human and animal contact, often in connection with ritualistic mutilation and murder. Given this history of highly aberrant sexual behavior, one may ask what the chances are of such a youngster's achieving a healthy psychosexual adjustment.

VI. ASSESSMENT OF DEVELOPMENT

Libido
Regarding Phase Development

In terms of ego development, Blanche was in latency; but in terms of libidinal development she was not a latency girl. The world of magic and witchcraft, in which sexuality is aggressive and aggression is sexual, had tampered with her phase development at several levels: phase dominance, age adequacy, and the maintenance of the highest level of phase development reached. The satanic cult did not tolerate frustration of libidinal drives, but focused on explicit need gratification without any restraint of basic primitive drives.

Assessment of Libidinal Fixation Points

When she was admitted to the hospital, Blanche had shown evidence of fixation in the oral sphere by her nightly oral-genital stimulation of her sister and oral sex with the family dog; the girls had been made to perform regular oral-genital stimulation on their mother. The extreme anxiety both girls manifested about eating meat certainly related to the cannibalistic activities of the cult within which they grew up. Evidence of anal fixation was manifested by Blanche's marked withholding of speech and interpersonal interaction. There is a diagnostic question as to whether her behavior showed willful withholding; indicated reaction formation; or entered the realm of pathological inhibition. Phallic concerns were demonstrated by her nightly bed-wetting, but these concerns had residues of oral and anal issues, so the bed-wetting could be understood as both a crying spell and a protest against her objects. Besides those oral and anal residues contaminating her phallic concerns, there were zonal confusions between front and back entrances, and great concern as to where she could be invaded bodily. This was demonstrated most vividly by Blanche's sleeping posture; crouched on her knees in a fetal position, she slept with one hand covering her genitals and the other covering her anus.

She was very prone to phallic, narcissistic wounds, could not compete, and could not tolerate her therapist's having other patients. However, toward the end of her stay in the hospital, shortly after she found her adoptive parents, hitherto subdued Oedipal wishes were unleashed. Previously, she had seemed oblivious to boy-girl relationships among her peers, but she now became infatuated with one of the more popular older boys in the hospital and asked staff how to greet him and how to assess his interest in her. Although she showed appropriate hesitation about interacting with him, she sought direction and support from members of the treatment team in learning how to approach the boy and communicate with him in a friendly way, and was able to follow through with the staff's guidance. She was quite philosophical in her acceptance of the boy's choice of an older girl, saying to staff members that she was too young at present to understand boyfriends. She also continued her close friendship with the teenage girl who was her rival, even after the two teenagers made their affection for one another public.

Clearly, work had been going on throughout her hospital stay to make this possible. Clinical material from her play therapy indicates that her involvement in this romantic triangle was not due to spontaneous entry into the Oedipal phase; her sessions were full of themes of competition with the female therapist and exploration of how the competition could be resolved. Having focused so much on this competition during her therapy, she was prepared when her adoption propelled her into the Oedipal area.

Libido Distribution

At the start of her stay in the hospital there was a tilt toward cathexis of self, but toward the end of her stay she seemed to reach a quantitative balance between self and other cathexes. Although initially preoccupied with self, when ready to leave the hospital she could reach out to others without fearing depletion of self-regard.

There is a diagnostic question about her initial self-orientation; specifically, was this self-focus due to disturbances caused by doubt about fitting into the world of her peers—a society of nonwitches? Or was it a disturbance of narcissism that inhibited her participation in group settings? Did she think she would disappear if she mixed with others? Would she lose her sense of self, disintegrate into nothingness if she merged with them? Was she afraid of contaminating the body person of others if she came in contact with them? The most plausible postulate may be that she was afraid of getting lost, as evidenced in her perseverative playing out of themes of lost-and-found, of moving in and out of existence, and of appearing and disappearing.

Her concern about disappearance of the self was exacerbated by the grip the world of magic had on her; the world of magic and the external world often seemed continuous. Her internal language of lost-and-found issues and fears of the disappearance of her own body-self were probably related to her objective world in which children were sacrificed by witches. Playmates could be seen on the playground one minute, but by the next they had disappeared—sacrificed and eaten.

At the start of her hospital stay Blanche laboriously and reluctantly made connections to others. She seemed tightly linked to her sister, who was unable to emerge from her psychosis to reciprocate. Blanche seemed to have had similarly intense bonds with "her two mothers," and had been deeply hurt by learning shortly after entering the hospital that her foster mother would not take her back. This news magnified the barriers she constructed between her self and others, and attempts to make contact with her resulted in the feeling that this child had enveloped herself in layer upon layer of psychic insulation that made her unavailable for human contact.

These barriers were broken primarily by her discovery of her therapist as a new objective. In this new relationship she moved from a completely walled-off posture toward the therapist to a period of voracious, insatiable appetite for her attention, and finally, to discovery and internalization of her analyzing functions. As treatment drew to a close, Blanche was tenacious and tireless in her curiosity about how families function, about her schoolwork, and about the world at large. Consistent with this shift came another, from a narcissistic object relation to a potential capacity for empathy.

Aggression

Although she had been guilty of fighting at the time of her referral, Blanche's generally quiet and timid disposition suggests a basic constitutional temperament not heavily endowed with aggressive drives. She engaged in aggressive behavior or threats of it when she felt threatened or provoked, as when her foster brother threatened to report her sexual activities. But when faced with the threatening presence of aggressive peers, she was extremely passive and showed no ability to defend herself. Her marked lack of assertiveness in the beginning of her hospital stay suggested a gross lack of development of the skills necessary for appropriate self-assertion. When told by those in authority to do something she disliked doing, she was typically compliant, but passively resisted completing these tasks.

She first expressed overt anger in therapy in the context of the transference, and gradually developed ways to do battle with her therapist in her play. Anger expression began in the form of a magical checkers game in which her checkers could fly around the room and capture the therapist's "men."

She then became capable of direct verbal expressions of anger at her sister, whose bizarre behavior had brought about the investigation that resulted in the girls' being uprooted from their biological mother's home. She expressed resentment at being confined to a hospital while Lucinda continued to enjoy the stability and commitment of the R's foster home. After quite a long time she was able to verbalize frustration with Lucinda's inability to return her love.

Anger at her biological mother was dealt with only in the context of the relationship with the therapist, but anger at the foster mother's perceived abandonment was eventually voiced very directly and appropriately. By the time Blanche was integrated into her new adoptive family she had openly questioned and tested almost every family rule and value until she was confident that the family structure was secure. She was spontaneous and direct with parents and siblings in the adoptive family at the time of her discharge from the hospital.

VII. EGO DEVELOPMENT

Physical Apparatus and Basic Psychological Functions

Physical apparatus subserving ego functions were intact.

Ego Functions

A psychological evaluation was completed six months after Blanche was admitted to the hospital. Her cognitive development was assessed with the Wechsler Intelligence Scale for Children—Revised and a learning disabilities battery. Her WISC-R subtest scaled scores were as follows:

Information	4	Picture Completion	10
Similarities	6	Picture Arrangement	9
Arithmetic	2	Block Design	8
Vocabulary	7	Object Assembly	9
Comprehension	7	Coding	9
(Digit Span)	(7)		

On substantially academic tests, such as those of word knowledge, mathematical ability, and acquired information, her performance was extremely poor. In contrast, she demonstrated average intellectual abilities in reasoning and problem-solving tests that did not contain school-related material. Her academic achievement was delayed by three years, and cognitive testing suggested problems with memory functions and a deficient attention span. In sum, she appeared to be a youngster with average intellectual potential who had not been able to respond to the academic stimulation of the classroom.

Projective testing revealed considerable guardedness in a youngster for whom interpersonal relations aroused overwhelming and unmanageable anxiety. Test data indicated a significantly distorted view of the interpersonal world, coupled with a strong tendency to avoid any sense of involvement or connectedness to others. Similarly, it appeared that Blanche was in the process of trying to install a rigid, entrenched avoidance of any direct experience of affect that was perceived as overwhelming.

She seemed to have given up attending to her environment or attempting to understand it. Instead, she seemed to be retreating from an external world she saw as chaotic, disorganized, and overwhelming. Her responses to the projective test material were indicative of excessive preoccupation with self at the expense of involvement with the world around her.

Ego Identification

Blanche was seen as heavily identified with her biological mother. She appeared to have thoroughly assimilated her mother's norms and aberrant culture. Evidence of this can be found in her continued sexual involvement with her sister and with animals while living with her foster family. Her threat to kill her foster brother if he spoke out about this forbidden activity is quite reminiscent of the visible reminders of death for those who might speak out about cult activities (e.g., the noose that hung in the girls' home.) Blanche did not speak negatively about her biological mother until the final months of therapy, when she was able at last to admit her mother's crimes and describe her as "too sick to live outside of a hospital."

Ego Reaction to Dangerous Situations

Blanche experienced danger from the outside world, which she perceived as a perilous place full of monstrous inhabitants always capable of murder and abuse. However, much more prominent in her work during her hospital stay was evidence of everpresent internal demons and monsters. Her fantasy play was full of tormenting, ghoulish monsters who could appear and disappear at any moment. She had little control over their appearance and disappearance. Also, she was plagued by fear of ghosts, particularly when she entered a bathroom. (Much of the mutilation of sacrificial victims' bodies apparently had occurred in the bathroom of her home.) She had horrible, agonizing nightmares nightly, and although they slowly became less frequent and intense, they never were altogether absent while she was in the hospital. The anguish of these nightmares was so overwhelming that she could not speak about them to nurses who would respond to her cries.

The predominant anxiety is an admixture of fear of annihilation, separation, object loss, and bodily damage. In her concern about separation from her biological mother, her intuition was that the separation would cause something terrible to happen to herself and to her mother; the locus of the danger was bodily damage.

Defense Organization

Defensive operation seemed to undergo significant changes in the course of her hospital stay. Massive repression was most evident initially. She presented as rigid, brittle, and unavailable, with no energy for the joys and activities in which the other children participated. Her failure to absorb any school material was striking; at the time of her admission she was illiterate.

Her use of compartmentalization was apparent. For example,

although she had sexual relations with her sister and with animals, she never attempted it with those outside the family, and she absolutely never talked about it. She compartmentalized her world into home and nonhome in many other respects, as reflected in differences in behavior at school and at home. She compartmentalized her play during her sessions, and made official announcements about the time for one kind of play to end and the time for another to begin. Her transitions between play activities were abrupt and formal rather than gradual.

Reaction formation became clear after she had been in the hospital for several months. She became the guardian of all animals; for example, when a caterpillar was found in some flowers on the ward, she immediately expressed great concern for its welfare in view of the approach of cold weather. She asked to adopt it, and make it a home in a tiny box in her room. Told that animal adoption was against hospital rules, and that a caterpillar could not live long or happily indoors, Blanche found a place for it in a quiet section of the garden outside the hospital, and went there often to try to find it and take it leaves to eat. As cold weather set in, she worried about its weaving a cocoon warm enough for its survival. Birds, squirrels, dogs, and cats were objects of similar attention on her part. And when describing the kind of new foster family she would like, she asked that it have a pet for her to love and care for.

Secondary Interference of Defense Activity with Ego Achievement

Not only was Blanche illiterate, but testing indicated problems in attention and concentration. Consistent with this was the test finding of failure to focus on and attempt to comprehend the world around her. All these findings point to the costly use of repression in shielding the youngster from actively inspecting, attempting to understand, and taking part in a world that was excessively confusing and dangerous. Her rigid compartmentalization of life experiences combined with social development. At home, and in the context of ritualistic sacrifices, she engaged in mutilation and murder, but was completely unprepared to participate actively and assertively in the normal give-and-take of everyday childhood relationships.

VIII. SUPEREGO DEVELOPMENT

Superego Proper

It appears that this child has negotiated the Oedipal conflict, and a relative sense of stability of introjects provides aim and direction.

The superego is structuralized, except that the introjects were quite aberrant. The fact that the introjects were so peculiar put Blanche in the position of potentially retreating into regressive positions. There is evidence of early damage in the internalizing process; she had internalized very dangerous introjects, but the stability of her superego gave her enough support that she had tried, albeit unsuccessfully, to report her mother's satanic activities to the authorities when she was five.

The superego was aim-giving throughout the treatment, but one cannot help wondering how she faced the murders and mutilation of animals and children without resorting to some form of cunning reassurance to appease the superego. The cult reinforced the bribery of the superego in many ways; for example, its murder victims were given new false names such as Moonbeam and Sunshine. Such names constituted, in effect, a denial of the victim as a person and rendered the victim unreal.

Blanche's play indicated that fathers are benign but ineffectual, while mothers are overwhelmingly powerful—close and nurturing, but potentially very dangerous and destructive. Also, mothers ask more of a child than a child is capable of. The mental construction of closeness and nurturing but also burdening was vividly expressed in the prominent pattern in Blanche's play in which a mare repeatedly forced a red and black robe like her own onto the back of her foal. Although the baby knew that the robe was a great gift, and that to wear it was an honor, it could not stand up under its weight. Its legs buckled, and it inevitably collapsed under the weight of the robe of honor.

The good news for Blanche was that in the first two-and-a-half years of her life while her father remained with the family, her mother was not known to have been involved in witchcraft activities.

The superego was effective, but the price was great: Blanche was too inhibited to learn in school until well after her removal from the cult, and she was shy and passive in social interaction.

The mechanisms for shoring up her superego, e.g., repression, reaction formation, were very characteristic of latency. However, in Blanche's case these mechanisms did not at first free her to learn and to socialize. But midway through treatment these constrictions were altered, and there was a great burst of intellectual activity, curiosity, and achievement that belonged to the latency phase.

This is a youngster who negotiated developmental stages effectively despite great obstacles to the progression of her development. However, there was always a nagging feeling that there was an island of madness within her that potentially could interfere with functioning.

Ego Ideals

By the middle of therapy Blanche's conscious aim was to become a psychologist. This was partly an identification with the therapist and partly an attempt to master her fears about her history, to give her traumatic past a decent burial. (If she could become a therapist she could then understand her past.) This wish to become a psychologist was growth-enhancing inasmuch as Blanche now put a premium on knowing, in sharp contrast to the pretreatment identification with her mother that underlay her threatening her foster brother with a knife to keep him from talking. The ego ideal of being a therapist thus became a means of disidentifying with her mother. The ideal thus was to be unlike the object.

IX. DYNAMIC AND STRUCTURAL ASSESSMENTS
(CONFLICTS)

There was external conflict, as when Blanche perceived that talking about the dangerous things she had seen would arouse her mother's wrath and bring on certain annihilation by the powerful cult.

There was internalized conflict-arousing guilt in Blanche, as when she would express fear of being hurt by hitchhikers; this fear of hitchhikers hurting her was a projection of her own aggressive impulses or a vicarious expression of the aggressive impulses of members of the witch coven. The source of this fear was really herself; it was she and her fellow witches who actually were likely to kill hitchhikers and street people. In perceiving hitchhikers as dangerous, she was really aware of the danger in herself.

X. GENERAL CHARACTERISTICS

Blanche could be irritable, but she never lashed out. Her frustration and tension tolerance was adequate and let her cope with weakening and rekindling anxiety in the course of treatment. She showed considerable sublimation potential in the form of a great burst of eagerness and yearning for involvement in learning. This suggested that she ultimately might not need pathological solutions. Although at the outset she gave the impression of wanting to avoid anxiety at any cost, by the end of her treatment it was clear that this early propensity never significantly impeded her functioning. Her progress suggested that a strong innate forward drive had withstood the madness of the witchcraft culture.

XI. DIAGNOSTIC STATEMENT

This is a girl who had achieved relative stability and sophistication in terms of ego and superego development. While her superego was structuralized before the massive trauma of cult involvement began, there is a question about possible physical abuse by her father during the first three years of Blanche's life. If it is true that the father abused her from time to time, we might surmise that internal images of those experiences had a perceptual identity with later forms of abuse seen in the coven. There may have been some proneness to neurosis or neuroticlike states resulting from her background of basic fantasies of pre-Oedipal beatings. With her subsequent involvement in the satanic cult, this child was certainly faced with a catastrophic outcome: the stalling of her development. She had a brittle ego, had difficulty in impulse control, and had only tentatively negotiated the Oedipus complex.

At the time of her discharge Blanche was in the process of being able to talk about, conceptualize, and understand her biological mother, but she continued to refuse open discussion of the activities of the cult. She was becoming more involved in the interpersonal world and made several good friends, but she was still quiet and shy. She was extremely modest about bathing and changing her clothing, loved school, and was fascinated by any new sort of learning.

Blanche was introduced to her new adoptive family by her therapist, and after they had visited her a few times in the hospital, she began joining them in their home for visits. After several weeks she became quite attached to her new family, and a date for her discharge was set.

Posthospital recommendations were for outpatient parent-guidance sessions, with none scheduled for Blanche in order to let her have time to rest and settle in to her remaining years of latency. The expectation was that the onset of puberty would reawaken many issues for her, and the family could plan for therapeutic assistance at that time.

One of the focal areas in the parent-guidance sessions was the support of the parents' upholding family norms. In contrast to her passive, compliant behavior on the ward, Blanche actively tested the adoptive family's rules, but she was met with firm and consistent limit-setting. She gradually achieved a comforting sense of the family's stability, and her efforts to test the limits subsided. The sessions also focused on supporting the parents' efforts to deal with Blanche's enuresis and nightmares. Although she had previously been unable to describe her nightmares to ward staff, she was able to talk to her adoptive mother, who readily provided support and comfort. After several weeks, nocturnal enuresis stopped, and the nightmares became less and less frequent.

The treatment team was surprised to learn that—in contrast to her characteristic reticence on the ward—soon after joining her adoptive family, Blanche began to recall particulars about the cult and to talk to her parents about it, sharing fears that it had caused her. Her adjustment to school and to her new siblings was very good, and she kept in touch with her sister.

Thus it appears that Blanche was able to use the stable support provided by her new family to achieve a healthy adjustment outside the hospital. She appears to have possessed the resources to cope with the many changes and traumas of her childhood, and at present her resources as an individual are combined with those of a loving, stable family to meet the challenges likely to come into her life at puberty.

CHAPTER 4

Family Narratives:
The Family and Treatment Contexts
of Polysymptomatic Behavior

PAUL E. TIETZE AND HOWARD F. STEIN

INTRODUCTION

This chapter addresses the question: How is one to proceed clinically when one is confronted by a seriously multisymptomatic family? It is a contribution to understanding and treating chaotic, underorganized, "acting out" families. It is often difficult enough to make etiological, diagnostic, and therapeutic sense of, say, schizophrenia or depression or diabetes when they come—at least ostensibly—as one diagnosis per family. We are all aware that an individual patient can have multiple problems and symptoms at the same time. How, then, is one to proceed when, in the same family, one discovers such an array of polysymptoms and diagnostic entities as depression, weight loss and physical deterioration, gastrointestinal disorder, attempted abduction of a child, marked recent weight gain, headache, and adolescent runaway—all within a single year (Wirshing and Stierlin 1985)?

In this chapter we describe a psychoanalytically informed, ethnographic, clinically acceptable ad hoc approach to the care of such a family (Stein 1982b, 1985b; Stein and Apprey 1985). This approach facilitates the emergence of the family's narrative, the story line that lies beneath and gives meaning to its symptomatology. Attending to the most obvious and potentially most dangerous symptoms, many clinicians read only the prologue of the family narrative. We affirm the value of listening to the clinical material at the level of the search for the organizing story (structural) line. At the same time, listening to and for a clinical story itself requires a common language. The writers draw upon classical psychoanalytic, object-relations, and structural theories for such a language of clinical investigation and intervention. This chapter describes the interplay of the family's and the clinician-authors' narratives, with special attention to the process of listening to the story in such a way as to find a version of it that expresses the reality of the family *and* the reality of the clinicians closely enough to allow useful interaction to occur. It is thus not only a chapter about "them" but also about how we learned to understand that onslaught of symptoms that was their family life.

At the level of process, the case to be described depicts and advocates treatment as a "holding environment" (Winnicott 1974) in which the family maelstrom of symptoms could be witnessed and ethnographically assessed (Stein and Pontious 1985), and its deeper, unifying meaning understood. We argue that, especially in the case of severe, multiproblem families, the presence of two people, one attending to biomedical issues and one to psychosocial, best enables this Winnicottian "holding" to occur. We likewise note a positive quality to the family members' symptoms over the course of treatment: i.e., symptoms, we shall argue, can signify improvement as well as pathology. At the more conceptual level this chapter is an exercise in systemic diagnostic thinking that may be useful when working with patients and families who present with an abundance of symptoms. We document that, in the primary-care based intervention that characterized the case that follows, *the process of uncovering the family story line with the family constitutes much (if not all) of the therapy itself* (Stein and Apprey 1985).

An approach similar to ours is that of Glenn (1984), who argues for the process of a negotiated diagnosis. This chapter takes a semiotic or meaning-centered (Geertz 1973; Kleinman 1980, 1983; Stein 1982a, 1984; Stein and Pontious 1985) approach to understanding family symptomatic behavior and intervention within that meaning system.

THE "FAMILY NARRATIVE" AS CLINICAL METAPHOR

We approach this case via the metaphor of narrative. During the course of this chapter, we hope to take the reader with us on an odyssey in an unfolding story line in which the writers also play a part. In this chapter we discuss a family with whom we have worked as family physician (PT) and behavioral scientist (HS) for a period of two years. We refer to them by the fictional name Craft. We describe a family narrative in which multiple symptoms in various members emerge as the "sections" progress. We also describe our role in the narrative, for we too have a role in the story line. It is a role that differs from the traditional, and at least official, biomedical narrative in which the physician perceives himself or herself to be the principal, if not the sole, "author" of the clinical narrative. Biomedicine emphasizes the need for the *doctor* to establish concisely the diagnosis of the patient, the ruling-in and ruling-out, of specific pathology. Physicians often think in terms of a closed biomedical package of content, whether or not that is appropriate to the reality of the family story line.

For many physicians and other American therapists, "doing" (i.e., intervention, action) is not only a professionally and culturally sanctioned mandate (Kluckhohn and Strodtbeck 1961; Parry 1984) but an inner compulsion as well (Stein 1985b). We often feel compelled to change others, and are buttressed in that feeling and ambition by professional authority. That can be a trap that makes one act peremptorily or prematurely. Our interventions in the family are in fact inseparable from our own process of learning about the family over many months as the family narrative progresses. Just as there is no such thing as an instant understanding of an individual patient's history, by working with family members and families as units we see *family* history unfold over time. In this chapter we show how, by understanding the family *process*, clinicians might alter a developing *pathological pattern* before the final, more severe, *expression* occurs.

We should say a word about our approach to understanding the influence of the family and the clinician upon health and the course of illness. The family is not a static, one-dimensional force or entity, but rather a multidimensional force field, so to speak (Spiegel 1971). By working with individual family members, one can affect familywide relationships (Bowen 1978). In attempting this, however, one must balance one's own biomedical linear thinking (which presupposes our control) with multidimensional, contextual thinking (in which we play a far more peripheral role than we may wish to acknowledge). By learning from the family its symptom manifestations and the meaning of these symptoms to family members and to the family as a whole, we learn how to intervene within their context and limits.

Biomedical practice tends to proceed on the assumption that with the initial patient encounter "You have to try to get everything at one time," that is, at least during the initial workup that may involve several visits and the collaboration of consultants. The very terms *complete history* and *complete physical* are part of the official medical vocabulary and mythology. The approach taken in this chapter departs markedly from this ideal, in part as a result of the recognition that, *in reality,* the ideal is untenable. The unfolding of the case makes clear that although the clinician would like to learn everything about the patient at once, much that is biomedically and psychosocially salient often cannot be obtained immediately. We get data, but often we do not—and cannot—know its significance in the larger clinical picture for a while.

This chapter is less a tale of differential diagnosis, prescriptions, and intervention than one of learning about the family as a guide to our intervention. Stated differently: here, as in classical psychoanalysis, the ethnographic "research" is intrinsic to the "intervention" or "therapy" itself. Therapy or clinical "action" does not strictly follow (sequentially) assessment and diagnosis. Instead, ongoing observation and participant observation coincides with clinical action for the purpose of continuously correcting it. Further, such contextual research is conducted *together with* one's subjects (patient, family) rather than exclusively "on" or "to" them. As the family narrative unfolds in the "holding environment" of the clinical relationship, the clinicians together with the family discover what is wrong and how to proceed from there.

Stated differently, as the drama unfolds, the clinician(s) help the family have the courage and tolerance to confront the story (often shared unconscious script) that underlies the assortment and timing of symptoms. Instead of striving to fulfill the maxim of "getting everything you need at once," we learned to strive to be able to listen attentively to the patient and her family so that meanings they shared with us would be adequately heard and could *then* be responded to. In the language of our metaphor, we permitted the family to narrate, even to enact, their story, in which they asked us—ever so cautiously—to intervene.

We now present a series of detailed accounts of specific clinical encounters ("sections" in the family narrative), followed by a discussion of overall family patterns.

SECTION 1: PRESENTATION OF "THE PROBLEM"

Martha brought sixteen-year-old Jenny Craft into the physician's office for evaluation of weight loss and fatigue. Martha was Jenny's stepmother and had been seen one year previously by the physician coauthor for tension headaches.

Jenny has lived in a rural Midwestern town for two years since coming from another area. She and her brothers (Eric and Bart) had come to this town to visit their father and stepmother. Their mother and father had divorced over the mother's sexual infidelity. The children never returned to their biological mother. Although she retained legal custody of these children, she knew their location and had not actively sought their return.

Martha dominated the interview, answering the questions directed at Jenny (who was quiet, appearing indifferent, even disinterested). Jenny did not protest Martha's intervention. In the waiting room prior to the interview, Martha had even filled out the patient history form for her stepdaughter. She put "16" for Jenny's *father's* age, the deeper significance of which became apparent much later in this family narrative.

Focusing on Jenny's symptoms through a biomedical lens, we found that she had lost greater than 15 percent of her weight (to her present ninety-nine pounds) and was apathetic about her weight loss. She had a domineering stepmother who was clearly being manipulated by her stepdaughter's eating behavior. Although she had not developed irregular menses and did not seem to have a "fat" body image, Jenny's eating behavior was clearly the focus of this medical visit and dialogue. An initial diagnosis of an eating disorder, perhaps early anorexia nervosa, was considered. Appropriate laboratory evaluation for common organic etiologies of weight loss proved negative, and Jenny was followed closely as an outpatient. Although the family was encouraged to attend later appointments, only Jenny and Martha came.

When Jenny failed to keep two appointments, then came to the clinic with an additional three-pound weight loss, she was hospitalized by the physician coauthor for a more extensive evaluation. Only a few days earlier her stepsister (Pamela), the youngest of the family, had been admitted to the hospital for acute lower abdominal pain that spontaneously resolved and for which no organic etiology was ever discovered.

While Jenny was in the hospital, discussion with her and her family began to bring "her problem" into context. The issues of greatest concern to Jenny centered around her feelings of having no control in (1) her home environment, (2) her relationship with a boyfriend (Michael), and (3) her own future plans. She found her choices increasingly being made by others. She liked to play basketball, but Martha insisted that she be a cheerleader. She wanted to become a secretary, but Martha wanted her to be a social worker (which Jenny thought would be "ok," although she could not de-

scribe what a social worker did). Her parents did not like her boyfriend. But when she seemed to make progress in their accepting
him, he would disappoint her by going out with old flames. Being
able to verbalize these issues seemed therapeutic for Jenny. She
gained weight steadily through her short hospitalization and was
discharged on Christmas Eve.

SECTION 2: OUT OF CONTROL

Following discharge from hospitalization, Jenny periodically
came into the office for weight checks. Although this had become
the "ticket" to the office, it was clearly no longer the central issue for
Jenny. She chose to use these visits as an opportunity to discuss her
boyfriend. Her relationship with him was literally on-again, off-
again daily. He would become drunk, roar off on his motorcycle,
take another girl out, then offer Jenny an engagement ring. Similarly, she alternately pleaded with her parents to accept him and
terminated their "steady" relationship. These same swings seemed
to pervade her home life as well.

Martha had placed Jenny in charge of her siblings and stepsib-
lings after school until her parents, who both worked, returned
home. Jenny's older biological brother, Eric, was peripheral to the
scene and planned to leave the household when he became eighteen (See genogram, figure 4.1). Eager to please her stepmother
and her father, Jenny accepted this responsibility but felt trapped
by it. Her lack of authority was heightened by her peer relationship
with her siblings whom she was to supervise. They misbehaved,
then talked her out of reporting their behavior to the parents. Her
parents, on discovering their misbehavior, chastised Jenny for not
reporting the problem to them. At this time Bart and Nick were
"peeping" when Pamela changed clothes, took a bath, or went to
the bathroom. Martha panicked, interpreting this as a developing
incestuous relationship while she was away at work. Ironically,
when, during the same period, Martha would berate Michael,
Jenny's boyfriend, she would encourage Jenny to "get along better"
with Charles, one of her sons.

When Jenny made a decision about anything, she was frequently
undermined by Martha. At one point, Jenny asked the physician
coauthor for birth control pills. She related that she and her stepmother had discussed the issue and Jenny didn't want to follow the
pattern of her stepmother's early (age sixteen) pregnancy. Subsequently, she discarded the birth control pills because her stepmother had admonished her that if she was on the pill, she couldn't

110

Figure 4.1   Genogram of the Craft family

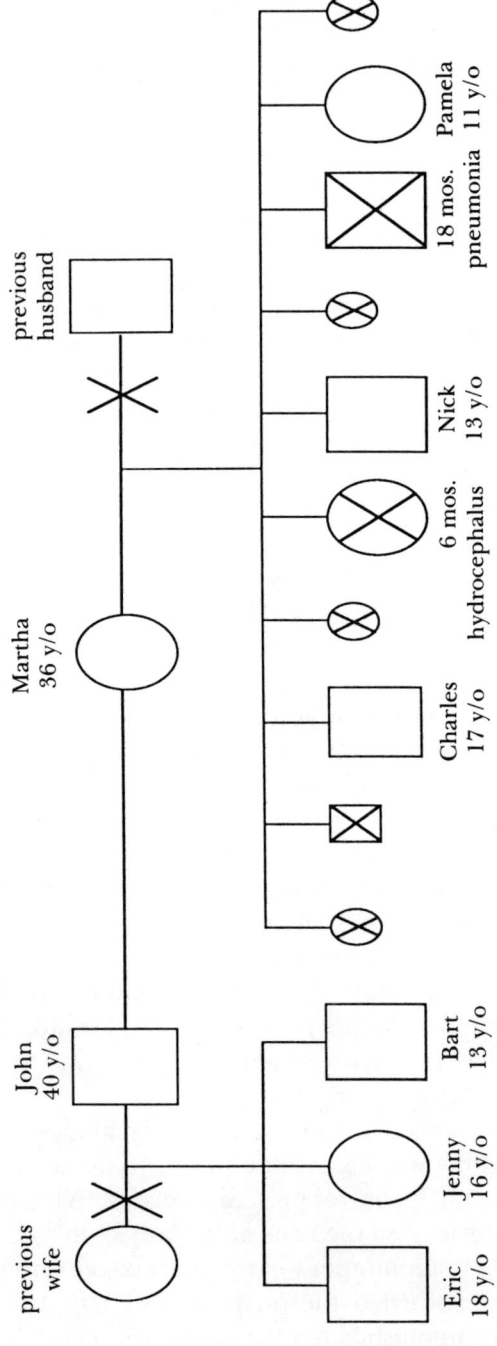

be trusted to abstain from sexual activity. Martha, who worked at a home for the handicapped, insisted that when Jenny became eighteen, she would have her stepdaughter declared mentally incompetent, and Jenny would therefore never be able to leave her present home.

SECTION 3: THE FAMILY AS PATIENT

Upon learning of the children's behavior that she labeled "incest," Martha quit her job at the home for the handicapped. Her husband, John, took a second job to compensate for the drop in family income. Discussions with the family revealed that the parents spent very little time together and didn't talk to each other. The parents described their life as hectic, since they were "doing all the work and self-sacrifice for the children." When asked what they anticipated doing when the children left home, they replied that they anticipated taking care of the grandchildren. Furthermore, they agreed it would be "impossible to go out on a date themselves," although previously Jenny had frequently watched the children for them in the early evening. Fear of intimacy, perhaps a reflection of earlier marriage difficulties and divorce, as well as the loss of children in the courts, and through stillbirths (Martha had had five stillbirths) pervaded their relationship.

During this family session, Jenny said to her parents, "I don't want to make you unhappy and I want to do my share of the work, but there is so much to do at home and I realize you need help." Previously, the expression of ambivalence about her domestic role had not been tolerable for Jenny or her parents. This was literally the most confrontive statement she had made since we had begun seeing the family. Mr. Craft (John) maintained emotional and physical distance from family and home, spending much of his time out working his cattle. Both Mr. Craft and his eldest son (Jenny's older brother), Eric, detached themselves from the world of home and attached themselves to the safer world of work and other men.

SECTION 4: RUNAWAY

On a late afternoon one spring day, the physician's office phone rang. John reported that Jenny had run away. Michael, Jenny's boyfriend, had picked up Jenny and Bart, her younger brother, and had taken them to the airport, hours away. John had received word they were to meet Jenny's biological mother there and to go live with her. John and Martha were on their way out the door, going to the airport to try to stop them.

The airport scene was bedlam. The police detained John and Martha and phoned Jenny to ascertain whether she had been kidnapped or was being held against her will. She had driven home from the airport with Michael. Subsequently, the police released John and Martha, who saw a tearful Bart dragged onto a waiting jet by his mother and stepfather. Because Jenny was sixteen, she had the legal right to decide with whom she would stay.

Jenny was seen in the emergency room that night. She was sobbing hysterically. She protested that she went to *see* her mother rather than to *leave* with her. When her mother made it clear that she wanted to take Jenny and Bart with her, Jenny fled. Bart felt he had been tricked into going to the airport to be delivered into his biological mother's hands. He had been in tears at being forcibly removed from the family. Jenny was upset that Bart felt betrayed by her, and she insisted it was never her intent that he be taken.

Martha was openly hostile to Jenny for making her relive the trauma of losing children. She now blamed Jenny for this most recent loss. John now attempted to act as a buffer between Jenny and Martha. He was encouraged that Jenny had made an active decision to stay with the family rather than going with her biological mother. Although he was upset that his son Bart was gone, this loss clearly did not have for him the profound impact or meaning it had for his wife. In the two weeks following the "runaway," there was a great deal of discussion of pain and loss: discussion of losing a daughter, losing a son, and of Martha's sense of displacement from her husband's attempts to intervene. Martha clearly was out of control (emotionally and in terms of running the family) and was extremely upset by it.

Slowly Martha's own intense sense of identification with her stepdaughter and her stepdaughter's script became evident to her. She saw her own adolescence relived. However, the older script was not being followed exactly. Separation between stepmother and stepdaughter was now occurring and this was a very painful process. Martha began to realize that her own script was not Jenny's. Her stepdaughter's inability to follow or to correct her stepmother's script was being played out before her.

SECTION 5: RECONCILIATION

Jenny and Martha came into the office after a trip to shop for a wedding dress, approximately one month after the runaway. Jenny was not pregnant but had made the decision to marry Michael. Martha accepted this decision. John, now emotionally removed again from the family, felt slighted that Michael had not asked him for Jenny's hand. He did not sanction the wedding, although he would not stand in Jenny's (or Martha's) way. He worried that Michael would not be a stabilizing influence in Jenny's life.

Michael and John were invited to the office, but only Michael came with Jenny and Martha. Michael sat quietly, physically removed from the stepmother and daughter in the office. He participated little in the discussion. He related that he wanted to be a good provider for Jenny.

On the next office visit the engagement had been broken off because Michael had again been seeing some old girlfriends. Jenny had returned the engagement ring and had decided not to see Michael any longer. In fact, she had gone out with a couple of other classmates and was surprised to find that several other boys were interested in going out with her. Jenny concluded that she had been wrong to concentrate her attention exclusively on Michael and resolved to continue dating other young men as well.

DISCUSSION

Working with this family felt like entering the landscape of a recurrent dream from which no one was permitted to awaken. Nothing dared change, yet so much had in fact changed for them all. It was only toward the end of the narrative in which we were involved that the multiple meanings of Jenny's initial symptoms became clear. Jenny had been left in charge of the household while her father and stepmother worked. Her role had been to keep the peace, which is to say, to keep the family together. Her father and stepmother had felt mutually isolated, and projected their feeling onto Jenny, fearing for *her* future. Part of her role had been to act as their buffer and to fill their emptiness. Her stepmother had reawakened her own poorly resolved adolescent conflicts and was reliving them in Jenny. The initial eating disorder and weight loss had been the family symptom of the dread of any changes.

Family members had been emotionally frozen in places at considerable distance from one another—John in the fields with his cattle, Martha a captive to the upholding of the home, Jenny striving to perfect herself in grades, school sports, and so forth. They kept together at the cost of enormous physical and emotional distance from each other, held by the dread of abandonment and the memory of repeated loss. Jenny tried to ingratiate herself with her stepmother, to placate her wishes, to propitiate her anger.

Jenny's biological mother, a dancer, had rarely been at home to care for her children before her divorce. Jenny, in turn, had become a virtual parent to her siblings and a dutiful homemaker to her father. She rarely saw her mother, whom she remembered had left very early and come home very late. After her parents' divorce, Jenny cared for her younger brother exclusively until the children moved in with their father. Her need to form a close relationship with a maternal figure was intense and compelling. Jenny said to us on one occasion, "When I came to live here, I guess I thought it was real important to get along; to have a mother" (referring to her then-new stepmother). Jenny, in turn, had identified with her step-mother's fear of marriage and pregnancy, and had defended herself by reaction formation against too closely allying herself with her biological mother's out-of-control sexuality (Wilson 1983). For both Jenny and her family, the fear of pregnancy vied with the wish to be pregnant. The quest for total control vacillated with spasms of being out of control.

For Jenny, the fear of disagreement overlay her dread of abandonment. Despite the great emotional and physical gulf between family members, there was a considerable blurring, if not a merging, of identities, resulting in contradictory communication. Martha related an incident in which she had been talking with Jenny about a problem. She had asked Jenny to express her own opinion, encouraging Jenny's independence. When Jenny finally replied somewhat angrily, Martha both verbally rebuked and slapped her—and regretted having done so ever since.

Similarly, as mentioned previously, Jenny had asked for birth control pills, and then later felt compelled to throw them away. Following her stepmother's comment that because Jenny had the pills, Martha could not trust Jenny to abstain from intercourse, Jenny felt the only way she could appear trustworthy was to throw the pills away—and risk becoming pregnant. At age sixteen, Jenny was precisely in the position her stepmother had been when she was sixteen: having to deny her own sexual intentions, having un-protected intercourse—and risking a pregnancy that would neces-sitate a forced marriage to please her parents. Jenny was unable to separate her own issues from those of her parents, and her parents were unable to separate from her.

During an early individual session, Jenny asked about the legality of her parents' stated intention to keep her at home after she was eighteen years old. She referred to her stepmother's verbal threat to declare her mentally incapable of caring for herself so she would be forced to continue to live with them. Although we quickly clarified the content issue of the legality matter, our meeting with her *as an individual* on several occasions was an attempt to honor the developmental issue of her own individuality and individuation. In fact, the underlying purpose of therapy was the individuation of all family members—conducted via those members who were willing to be in treatment.

Because of their dread of the past, the family unwittingly repeated it. Jenny's longtime on-again, off-again boyfriend was said to "sneak around," as her natural mother was remembered to have done. Moreover, her stepmother had been forced to marry at age sixteen (due to pregnancy and family pressure), just as Jenny had been feeling somehow compelled to marry during this year. Meanings such as these emerged from our participant observation that led us to listen carefully to the family narrative.

During the initial appointment at the family-medicine clinic, Martha had mistakenly written on the initial patient-encounter questionnaire that her stepdaughter's father's age was sixteen, when he was, in fact, forty. We later learned, after numerous individual and family sessions, that Martha had been forced at sixteen to marry the sixteen-year-old young man by whom she had become pregnant. Moreover, Jenny, now sixteen, was in a relationship with a young man of sixteen. In time it became clear that Martha feared her stepdaughter would repeat what she had done at the same age. The "error" on the patient-encounter form was in fact a parapraxis, one that gave further credence to our impression of the stepmother's projective identification with her stepdaughter. Again, practitioners often acquire clinical facts, but have little idea of their meaning until much later.

At the family session immediately following the brief runaway episode—attended by Jenny, her father, and her stepmother—the atmosphere was heavy with foreboding and guilt. Everyone was silent. The stepmother, chain-smoking, began to cry quietly, saying that she felt she had lost something or someone had died. She was asked: "Who died?" She replied: "Myself, I feel like I died; I feel that I lost myself." She added after a period of silence, "I feel like I have lost my daughter" (reflecting a blurring of her identity with Jenny's). Jenny said tearfully that she felt "guilty for running away." Her stepmother sobbed heavily. The therapist turned to her, and she fended him off saying, "No, don't ask me to say anything. . . . I'd just like to run away. I wish to God I had the courage to run away." The consultant pointed out that this is exactly what Jenny had done, that Jenny had acted as Martha's proxy.

During the remainder of the interview, the husband and wife started talking *with each other* about their problems: Martha wanted to be more assertive, yet felt she had to acquiesce; wanted John to stand up to her, not be a "yes man," yet not to subvert her correcting the children. They talked more openly about their disagreements.

Earlier the parents had recounted their pain of having lost children (John losing custody in court battles and Martha losing children in childbirth and in infancy). They dreaded further loss—the burden of the past that was to have been eased through Jenny's loyalty. Yet they both gradually came to acknowledge their own disloyal feelings. What Jenny had done against the family's wishes but in their behalf, her stepmother could only now wish aloud for herself.

In some of the final sessions, the stepmother began to affirm that there were worse things in life than feeling alone; she had survived this feeling before and could do it again. Whereas before she had felt compelled to make the perfect home for her husband in order to preserve the marriage, she now resolved that, for instance, if their roof continued to leak, she would not feel compelled to fix it alone, but would risk leaving it to him. For the first time in a year of family sessions, the stepmother appeared neatly dressed and radiant and spoke with dignity (rather than with accusation or self-accusation).

Around this same time, Jenny and her boyfriend-fiancé again broke their engagement and began dating others. Jenny found a job she liked that did not interfere with her schoolwork. We know little of the outcome for Jenny's father, for he did not attend the last sessions in order to tend to the harvest in late spring/early summer (Stein 1982a). Although we had tried to include him in treatment many times, he continued to use his work to keep his emotional distance from the family.

The prevalence of problems of control and boundaries in families such as the Crafts can be understood not only through their interactions but also through examining the meanings their relationships had for the family participants. What can the symptom choice—e.g., weight loss, running away, etc.—tell us about the family symbolism: in particular, how members internally represent themselves and each other? And how does this further inquiry influence *our* perception of the symptom and our approach to treatment? Summarizing a considerable literature on the defense mechanism of projective identification, first formulated by Melanie Klein (1946), Sander writes that:

Just as a child in the rapprochement crisis may defend against further separation by regressive clinging and other manipulations of significant others, families of borderline patients also defend against further differentiation and separation by a host of interpersonal maneuvers. They, for example, limit self-object differentiation by a defensive delineation of the other that tries to deny the realistic parts of the other [clearly illustrated by the response of Jenny's stepmother to Jenny]. This process first described by Melanie Klein [1946] as projective identifications had been further reviewed and discussed by Jaffe [1968] and Robbins [1976]. Shapiro and his colleagues frequently found this mode of "defensive" perception and behavior in the families they studied [Zinner and Shapiro 1972]. (1979:130)

Projective identification thus regulates relationships and inner states at the same time. Our argument is, not that Jenny is definitively borderline, but rather that she and her family have used "interpersonal maneuvers" to stave off painful emotional separation. Klein states: "Identification by projection implies a combination of splitting off parts of the self and projecting them onto (or rather into) another person" (1955:311–12). It is "the feeling of identification with other people, because one has attributed qualities or attitudes of one's own to them" (1955:311). In families, the symptom-bearer is often the person who officially acts out functions for the other family members with whom this person is projectively identified. Serving as a defense against separation anxiety, the mechanism represents an inability to let go. The family deposits, as it were, their disavowed parts and impulses into another who, for personal reasons, is willing to serve as the family repository. In their seminal paper that examined projective identification as a regulator in families with borderline adolescents, Zinner and Shapiro wrote that:

> Projective identification is an activity of the ego, which among its effects, modifies perception of the object and, in a reciprocal fashion, alters the image of the self. These conjoined changes in perception influence and may, in fact, govern behavior of the self toward the object. Thus, projective identification provides an important conceptual bridge between an individual and interpersonal psychology, since our awareness of the mechanism permits us to understand specific interaction *among* persons in terms of specific dynamic conflicts occurring within individuals. (1972:523)

Jenny's eating problems were simultaneously a personal and a family defense. Our difficulty in working with her and her family lay partly in our inability, for quite some time, to identify *what* the underlying problems were and *where* they were located. For a while, all we could recognize was the pall of sameness that fogged over the invisible sea of despair. In addition to Jenny's "primary" and "secondary" gain, we came to recognize the family's "tertiary" gain of defense achieved in and through her.

Sander writes that:

> Defenses, by definition, defend against unacceptable unconscious impulses, affects, wishes, or fantasies. They protect the ego against instinctual demands and for the most part are intrapsychic in their operation, though they all have some interpersonal consequences. . . . As drive theory becomes more integrated with object-relations theory, the concept of defense needs expansion to include its interpersonal ramifications. Perhaps it would be more accurate to speak of such ego activities as serving (1) defensive functions for the individual and (2) equilibrating, adaptive, or maladaptive functions for a family or group. (1979:129)

Jenny's eating disorder and running away served simultaneous personal and family systemic defensive functions—the brief running away being more "progressive" than the weight loss and physical deterioration. Her running away was not only symptomatic of family wishes but was tearfully envied by her stepmother. The running-away episode, in our interpretation, represented a thawing of the frozenness of her symptoms as a family defense.

How did Jenny's weight loss function? It can be seen as a condensation and compromise formation for Jenny and her family, Jenny as the official *symptom-bearer* of her family. Through her weight loss Jenny (1) expressed her longing to be perfect (asexual) and thereby to merit approval from her stepmother; (2) expressed her wish to avoid repeating the patterns of her mother and stepmother (sneaking around sexually, early pregnancy, and marriage) and her simultaneous identifications with mother and stepmother; (3) expressed her flight from adolescence, womanhood, and motherhood; (4) expressed her longing to remain an asexual child, daddy's girl, and stepmommy's dutiful daughter; (5) expressed forbidden aggression toward her parents in the masochistic form of punishing them by punishing (depriving) herself; (6) exerted her independence while remaining totally dependent upon her father and stepmother; (7) preserved the integrity of the family and embodied its separation anxiety; and (8) was punished for her burgeoning sexuality and thereby vindicated the family (Freud 1919).

In short, through Jenny's eating behavior and weight loss, the family's conflicts over separation and sexuality were played out and controlled. And in many respects, in choosing these as her symptoms, Jenny became a defensive bulwark on behalf of the family: her predominant symptom, metaphor for her identity, was simultaneously hers and theirs. In *her* symptom lay *their* destiny; and conversely.

CULTURAL ISSUES

Thus far, we have discussed Jenny's eating disorder and related behavior in individual and family contexts. In this section we briefly consider it in the wider cultural context of such widespread American eating disorders as anorexia nervosa, bulimia, overeating, and obesity. Although it is debatable whether Jenny's eating problems could be stretched on the taxonomic procrustean bed into the diagnosis anorexia nervosa, we shall culturally consider her problems as if they were somewhat related to the classical picture. Jenny's obsession with thinness and weight can be understood as part of a highly prevalent culturally stylized pattern if not a culture-bound syndrome. (For examples of the extensive and heated debate over the concept of culture-bound syndromes, see Beiser 1987; Burton-Bradley 1983; Hahn 1985; Johnson 1987; Kapur 1987; Kirmayer 1987; Kleinman 1987; Landy 1987; Langness 1981; Lock 1987; Prince 1985; Prince and Tcheng-Laroche 1987; Simons 1987; and Stein 1985a). Discussing anorexia nervosa in terms of "the cultural determinants of the syndrome in the form of values, beliefs, and symbol systems," psychiatrist Raymond Prince observes that: "As Westerners, we all experience first hand the powerful anorexic influences that are currently playing upon us, particularly upon the Western female. The slim, youthful body is beautiful and healthy; the fat person is slovenly, ugly, prone to disease and lacks self-discipline. Less conscious perhaps are the forces calling for the equality of the sexes, and the implied rejection of female contours and motherhood. A significant proportion of women and men concern themselves inordinately with dieting and exercising" (1985:119).

The late psychoanalyst and anthropologist George Devereux (1980) has contributed notably to the understanding of the psychocultural dynamics of cultural elaborated patterns such as *koro* (the fear and belief that the penis is retracting and that the afflicted person will die; widespread in China) and *amok* (prodromal brooding, followed by homicide, persistence of homicidal urge, and resolution with amnesia; widespread in Malaysia, the Philippines, and

Papua New Guinea), a framework that can be applied to anorexia nervosa as well. When a culture has standard "type conflicts," that culture over time elaborates a set of standardized defenses and solutions for these conflicts. "The cultural normalization of such disorders not only allows them to be used as models for individuals who for some reason are psychically disturbed; it also permits the same abnormality to be triggered by a wide variety of different stimuli" (1980:29). Precisely because of the "cultural conformism" of the symptom patterns of patients with these conventional syndromes, clinicians are often misled into "underestimating the seriousness of their fundamental pathology" (1980:40). Moreover, "what underlies an ethnic [cultural] disorder is not simply the specific psychodynamic configuration that determines its etiology, but a particular ethnic [cultural] character as well—one so conditioned as to allow the subject to rid himself of a number of diversified subjective problems by means of one and the same complex of symptoms" (1980:45). Finally, the widely patterned pathology serves as a commentary on the cultural system it violates as it exaggerates: "In every ethnic [cultural] disorder it is chiefly the pattern, rather than any one of its component elements, that is abnormal, and this abnormality is, in a way, a caricature of the total culture pattern" (1980:47). Using a systemic model, Selvini Palazzoli likewise argues that "the culture in which a symptom develops has a determining effect upon the appearance of the symptom itself; each specific culture furnishes a certain type of discomfort the means to express itself" (1985:204).

In two books, *The Obsession: Reflections on the Tyranny of Slenderness* (1981) and *The Hungry Self: Daughters and Mothers, Eating, and Identity* (1985), Kim Chernin identifies culturewide psychodynamic themes that find expression in female thinness: e.g., symbolic matricide, reaction formations against devouring/being overwhelmed by the mother, wishes for merger with the mother, compulsive dieting as an attempt to separate from the mother but attesting to the failure of the attempt, wishes to remain childlike and masculine. Yates, Leehey, and Shisslak (1983) in their analysis of compulsive "runners" and "joggers," and Stein (1982c, 1982d, 1982e) in a series of papers on the cultural significance of the "wellness" or "fitness" movement, have argued that the dynamics, albeit not the extremes, of anorexia nervosa are present in mainstream American life and in its body-image ideals. Highly prevalent and painstakingly stylized pathologies attest to and express conflicts shared by great numbers of officially normal persons in the culture (Henry 1963; Mead 1947;

Stein 1985a). Just as the symptom-bearing adolescent with an eating disorder is the (primary) identified patient in the family discussed in the case above and in countless families with anorectic members, likewise do anorectics *as patients and as exemplars alike* function as "social cynosures" (La Barre 1956), types of persons who attract a great deal of attention within the society.

Writing of widespread eating disorders as cultural metaphor, Scheper-Hughes and Lock note that

> Crawford (1984) has interpreted the eating disorders and distortions in body image expressed in obsessional jogging, anorexia, and bulimia as a symbolic mediation of the contradictory demands of postindustrial American society. The double-binding injunction to be self-controlled, fit, and productive workers, and to be at the same time self-indulgent, pleasure-seeking consumers is especially destructive to the self-image of the "modern," "liberated" American woman. Expected to be fun-loving and sensual, she must also remain thin, lovely, and self-disciplined. Since one cannot be hedonistic and controlled simultaneously, one can alternate phases of binge eating, drinking, and drugging with phases of jogging, purging, and vomiting. Out of this cyclical resolution of the injunction to consume and to conserve is born, according to Crawford, the current epidemic of eating disorders (especially bulimia) among young women, some of whom literally eat and diet to death. (1987:26)

It would appear that anorexia nervosa (and other eating disorders), like other social forms—from folktale to poem to novel— simultaneously offers "models" for the channeling or expression of widely shared problems *and* for the symbolizing of more idiosyncratic and familiosyncratic conflicts (a point that Stein has recently made concerning American alcoholism, 1985a). In a historical overview of anorexia nervosa, Charles C. Hogan notes that "All the contributors to [*The Fear of Being Fat*, edited by C. Philip Wilson, 1983] are impressed with the heterogeneity of anorexic patients— by the great dynamic, structural, and genetic variability under the coating of a relatively uniform symptomatology" (1983:2). Wilson repeatedly shows how "Conflicts from every developmental phase can be repressed and displaced onto the fear of being fat" (1983:18). Stated differently, the presence of a culturewide form for the expression of conflicts means that persons/families having a common denominator of conflicts will not have to "improvise" with solutions; it also means that these cultural forms (i.e., widely accepted symptom patterns) become available for use by individuals and families as vehicles for more personal, "deeper" issues. As a culturally stylized disorder, anorexia nervosa (like other eating disorders) performs a homeostatic function simultaneously at the personality, family, and cultural levels—a fact that helps to account for its refractoriness in treatment.

What all this means for the American practitioner of any clinical specialty or theoretical proclivity is that the more difficult a pattern of behavior and meaning is to *contain*—the more large numbers of people participate in it—the more refractory it will be to treatment because so many people (including well-intentioned therapists) are themselves part of the disorder. Treatment can subtly collude as unconscious resistance to comprehending the disorder (see Stein 1984). The utility of the ethnographic approach we have taken in this "family narrative" of eating problems and other symptoms in context is that it facilitates the emergence of the story behind the story. Through the parallax of time and clinical relationship, a wider and deeper knowledge of the pathological process, and how to intervene in it, is possible. Through our work with Jenny and her family we have learned that—simultaneously at individual, family, and cultural levels—the eating disorder served as a powerful compromise formation, both revealing and concealing, expressing and displacing, a source of pain and—costly—pleasure.

CONCLUSION

In several medical and social science disciplines, there is already a prodigious literature on eating disorders, incest, voyeurism, runaway adolescents, and depression. Even within the burgeoning family-therapy and family-medicine literature, there is the tendency to view these symptoms (and others) as discrete clinical entities. Although for heuristic purposes and emergency interventions such a view is necessary, it tends to falsify the reality of the ebb and flow of family relationships and meanings. This chapter has explored the interplay of symptom (or disease) choice and family relationships over time: i.e., from the first time the family physician coauthor saw the stepmother as patient to a period two years later when the physician-coauthor completed his residency. This latter event coincided with the time that the clinic business office peremptorily terminated the family because of unpaid bills—a fact that in turn directs our attention to extrafamilial constraints upon the family and treatment system. There is often far more beyond our clinical control than we wish to acknowledge. Within these constraints, we were able to gain an understanding of the deeper order beneath the surface chaos (Nurnberg and Shapiro 1983; Reiss 1981).

Documenting the expression of the family patterns in symptom formation over time, we have argued that the unfolding of symptoms represents the emerging of underlying shared issues, a family isomorph with the "return of the repressed" and the "rendering of the unconscious conscious" in psychoanalytically oriented therapy. Noting a progression of symptoms from weight loss and eating disturbance to running away, we further suggested that, paradoxically, under certain conditions, one can and must view pathology as improvement. Consistent with a systems view of the family *and* treatment process, we also discussed what it was like to work with this family. For, if the process of clinical intervention can be viewed as a narrative, that unfolded over time, we in fact coauthored a story line that facilitated the emergence of the deeper family narrative.

In this chapter we have likewise urged that in work with families, one must be familiar enough with and profoundly moved by the family narrative in order to know how and when to intervene in it. It is, finally, not enough for the therapists to know only the "text" of the family narrative. It is necessary for the therapists to embark on the even more disquieting journey of comprehending the meaning of that narrative—a task that requires one to look inward in behalf of the family (akin to "regression in the service of the other," Olinick 1969). One uses one's own emotional "resonance" to understand the family and to help them understand themselves and to change. Thus, paradoxically, the therapist who best *leads* is one who can also *follow.*

REFERENCES

Beiser, M. 1987. Commentary on "Culture-bound syndromes and international disease classifications," by R. Prince, and F. Tcheng-Laroche. *Culture, Medicine and Psychiatry* 11(1):29–33.

Bowen, M. 1978. *Family therapy in clinical practice.* New York: Jason Aronson.

Burton-Bradley, B. 1983. Transcultural psychiatry. *Medical Education International Ltd.*, pp. 1625–26.

Chernin, K. 1981. *The obsession: Reflections on the tyranny of slenderness.* New York: Harper and Row.

———. 1985. *The hungry self: Daughters and mothers, eating and identity.* New York: Times Books.

Crawford, R. 1984. A cultural account of health: Self control, release, and the social body. In *Issues in the political economy of health care,* edited by J. McKinlay. London: Tavistock.

Devereux, G. 1980. Normal and abnormal. In his *Basic problems of ethnopsychiatry,* translated by B. M. Gulati and G. Devereux, 3–71. Chicago: University of Chicago Press (orig. 1956).

Freud, S. 1919. "A child is being beaten": A contribution to the study of the origin of sexual perversions. In *The standard edition of the complete psychologi-*

cal works of Sigmund Freud (SE) 17, translated by J. Strachey, 175–204. London: Hogarth Press, 1955.

Geertz, C. 1973. *The interpretation of cultures: Selected essays.* New York: Basic Books.

Glenn, M. 1984. *On diagnosis: A systemic approach.* New York: Brunner/Mazel.

Hahn, R. A. 1985. Culture-bound syndromes unbound. *Social Science and Medicine* 21(2):165–71.

Henry, J. 1963. *Culture against man.* New York: Vintage Books/Random House.

Hogan, C. C. 1983. Introduction. In *The fear of being fat: The treatment of anorexia nervosa,* edited by C. P. Wilson, 1–5. New York: Jason Aronson.

Jaffe, D. S. 1968. The mechanism of projection: Its dual role in object relations. *International Journal of Psycho-Analysis* 49:662–77.

Johnson, T. M. 1987. Premenstrual syndrome as a Western culture-specific disorder. *Culture, Medicine and Psychiatry* 11(3):337–56.

Kapur, R. L. 1987. Commentary on "Culture-bound syndromes and international disease classifications," by R. Prince and F. Tcheng-Laroche. *Culture, Medicine and Psychiatry* 11(1):43–48.

Kirmayer, L. J. 1987. Review of *Culture-bound syndromes/folk illnesses of psychiatric and anthropological interest,* edited by R. C. Simons and C. C. Hughes. *Transcultural Psychiatric Research Review* 24(4):275–83.

Klein, M. 1946. Notes on some schizoid mechanisms. *International Journal of Psycho-Analysis* 27:99–110.

———. 1955. On identification. In *New directions in psycho-analysis,* edited by M. Klein, P. Heimann, and R. Money-Kyrle, 309–45. New York: Basic Books.

Kleinman, A. 1980. *Patients and healers in the context of culture: An exploration of the borderland between anthropology, medicine, and psychiatry.* Berkeley and Los Angeles: University of California Press.

———. 1983. The cultural meanings and social uses of illness: A role for medical anthropology and clinically oriented social science in the development of primary care theory and research. *The Journal of Family Practice* 16(3):539–45.

———. 1987. Culture and clinical reality: Commentary on "Culture-bound syndromes and international disease classifications," by R. Prince and F. Tcheng-Laroche. *Culture, Medicine and Psychiatry* 11(1):49–52.

Kluckhohn, F., and F. Strodtbeck. 1961. *Variations in value orientations.* Evanston, Ill.: Row Peterson.

La Barre, W. 1956. Social cynosure and social structure. In *Personal character and cultural milieu,* edited by D. G. Haring, 535–46. New York: Syracuse University Press.

Landy, D. 1987. Review of *Culture-bound syndromes/folk illnesses of psychiatric and anthropological interest,* edited by R. C. Simons and C. C. Hughes. *Medical Anthropology Quarterly* 1(3):345–47.

Langness, L. L. 1981. Abstract of "Falling out: A diagnostic and treatment problem viewed from a transcultural perspective," by H. H. Weidman [Social Science and Medicine 13 B (1979):95–112]. *Transcultural Psychiatric Research Review* 18(3):216–19.

Lock, M. 1987. DSM-III as a culture-bound construct: Commentary on "Culture-bound syndromes and international disease classifications," by

R. Prince and F. Tcheng-Laroche. *Culture, Medicine and Psychiatry* 11(1): 35–42.

Mead, M. 1947. The concept of culture and the psychosomatic approach. *Psychiatry* 10:57–76.

Nurnberg, H. G., and L. M. Shapiro. 1983. The central organizing fantasy. *Psychoanalytic Review* 70(4):493–503.

Olinick, S. L. 1969. On empathy and regression in the service of the other. *British Journal of Medical Psychology* 42:41–49.

Parry, K. K. 1984. Concepts from medical anthropology for clinicians. *Physical Therapy* 64(6):929–33.

Prince, R. 1985. The concept of culture-bound syndromes: Anorexia nervosa and brain-fag. *Social Science and Medicine* 21(2):197–203.

Prince, R., and F. Tcheng-Laroche. 1987. Culture-bound syndromes and international disease classifications. *Culture, Medicine and Psychiatry* 11(1):3–19.

Reiss, D. 1981. *The family's construction of reality.* Cambridge: Harvard University Press.

Robbins, M. 1976. Borderline personality organization: The need for a new theory. *Journal of the American Psychoanalytic Association* 24:381.

Sander, F. M. 1979. *Individual and family therapy: Toward an integration.* New York: Jason Aronson.

Scheper-Hughes, N., and M. M. Lock. 1987. The mindful body: A prolegomenon to future work in medical anthropology. *Medical Anthropology Quarterly* 1(1):6–41.

Selvini Palazzoli, M. 1985. Anorexia nervosa: A syndrome of the affluent society. *Transcultural Psychiatric Research Review* 12(3):199–205.

Simons, R. C. 1987. A feasible and timely enterprise: Commentary on "Culture-bound syndromes and international disease classifications," by R. Prince and F. Tcheng-Laroche. *Culture, Medicine and Psychiatry* 11(1):21–28.

Spiegel, J. 1971. *Transactions: The interplay between individual, family, and society.* New York: Science House.

Stein, H. F. 1982a. The annual cycle and the cultural nexus of health care behavior among Oklahoma wheat farming families. *Culture, Medicine and Psychiatry* 6(1):81–99.

———. 1982b. The ethnographic mode of teaching clinical behavioral science. In *Clinically applied anthropology: Anthropologists in health science settings,* edited by N. Chrisman and T. Maretzki, 61–82. Boston: D. Reidel.

———. 1982c. "Health" and "wellness" as euphemism: The cultural context of insidious draconian health policy. *Continuing Education for the Family Physician* 16(3):33–44.

———. 1982d. Neo-Darwinism and survival through fitness. *The Journal of Psychohistory* 10(2):163–87.

———. 1982e. Wellness as illusion. *Delaware Medical Journal* 54(11):637–41.

———. 1984. "Misplaced persons": The crisis of emotional separation in geographical mobility and uprootedness. *The Journal of Psychoanalytic Anthropology* 7(3):269–92.

———. 1985a. Alcoholism as metaphor in American culture: Ritual desecration as social integration. *Ethos* 13(3):195–235.

————. 1985b. *The psychodynamics of medical practice: Unconscious factors in patient care.* Berkeley and Los Angeles: University of California Press.

Stein, H. F., and M. Apprey. 1985. *Context and dynamics in clinical knowledge,* vol. 1 of the Series in Ethnicity, Medicine, and Psychoanalysis. Charlottesville, Va.: University Press of Virginia.

Stein, H. F., and J. M. Pontious. 1985. Family and beyond: The larger context of noncompliance. *Family Systems Medicine* 3(2):179–89.

Wilson, C. P., ed. 1983. *The fear of being fat: The treatment of anorexia nervosa and bulimia,* with the assistance of C. C. Hogan and I. L. Mintz. New York: Jason Aronson.

Winnicott, D. W. 1974. *Through paediatrics to psychoanalysis: The collected papers of D. W. Winnicott.* New York: Basic Books (orig. 1958, Tavistock).

Wirshing, M., and H. Stierlin. 1985. Psychosomatics I. Psychosocial characteristics of psychosomatic patients and their families. *Family Systems Medicine* 3(1):6–16.

Yates, A., K. Leehey, and C. M. Shisslak. 1983. Running—An analogue of anorexia? *The New England Journal of Medicine* 308(5):251–55.

Zinner, J., and R. L. Shapiro. 1972. Projective identification as a mode of perception and behavior in families of adolescents. *International Journal of Psycho-Analysis* 53:523–30.

Chapter 5

Illness Experience and Disease Process: An Ethnographic Study of a Disabled Individual

HOWARD F. STEIN AND LARRY ROEDIGER

INTRODUCTION (Stein)

The chapter that follows is the product of a graduate seminar on human behavior in occupational medicine that I led in the autumn of 1982. The chapter, like the orientation of the course, is largely ethnographic, which is to say that the goal is to understand how individuals experience, organize, and assign meaning to the world. In contemporary Western medical settings, this is tantamount to supplementing a biomedical account of the disease process with one of the illness experience (see Kleinman 1980, Stein 1980, Eisenberg and Kleinman 1981). As the reader will shortly see, however, the causal arrow does not so swiftly fly from "disease" to "illness." The two constitute a unitary system with implications for one another. In his ethnographic study of a disabled Southwestern male, Larry Roediger, a Physician's Associate (P.A.), discovered how an abundance of disease entities "fit" in a perfect yet sinister way with the patient's and family's organization around his illnesses as their way of life. He also hints at how the health care system—here, the Veterans Administration hospital—inadvertently and insidiously became interwoven into the fabric of the patient's and family's ethos: they simultaneously were compelled to care for him *and* to fail him (see also Stein 1982a).

Some years ago I had made a home visit to this patient at the request of a clinician in the back clinic of a Southwestern Veterans Administration (VA) hospital. I was to help evaluate the patient's request for a mechanical lift from his driveway to his door. It was explained to me that he was 100 percent disabled, and that he had virtually no range of motion in his arms. Yet during an hour's lively conversation, he proceeded to remove the tight halo brace from his neck, and to adjust his sling. At his bequest, his wife gave me a tour of their home—a veritable private hospital: hospital beds, massive wheelchairs, etc. Medical paraphernalia sprawled throughout the house; not a single area was exempt from its influence. While he had been a patient of my colleague for nearly a decade, little was known about the relationship between his diseases and his life. This single home visit could only begin to fill in the gaps.

As the seminar began in the early fall of 1982, Mr. Roediger expressed some interest in working with the patient and family as his project in occupational medicine and human behavior. My colleague in the back clinic telephoned the patient's home to pave the way—only to have the patient's wife sob to him that her husband had recently turned heavily to alcohol. On religious grounds the patient had previously condemned alcohol use and during one home visit had denied, in the presence of his wife, ever drinking. With tape recorder in hand, Mr. Roediger made several visits to the patient's home and to the homes of the patient's children. The result is Mr. Roediger's case study of the meaning of illness in this patient's life—and of how countless others have gravitated to participate in and confirm that meaning.

Following the case presentation by Larry Roediger, I offer a brief commentary.

THE ETHNOGRAPHY (Roediger and Stein)

Work and Social History

John Calvin Smithson is a fifty-seven-year-old male Caucasian born in southern Oklahoma. Mr. Smithson has an Anglo-Saxon ethnic background. His parents were farmers, but moved to Dallas, Texas, due to the Great Depression of the 1920s. Mr. Smithson's father had not been able to make any money farming during the 1920s, so he moved his family in order to find employment. A brief description of John's life and work history can be found in figure 5.1.

John C. Smithson obtained a high school education while working part-time, as a result of his father's request that his son learn "a trade." John started working for a plumbing business as a member of a crew that installed bathrooms for an affiliated building contractor. He continued this part-time work until he graduated from high school.

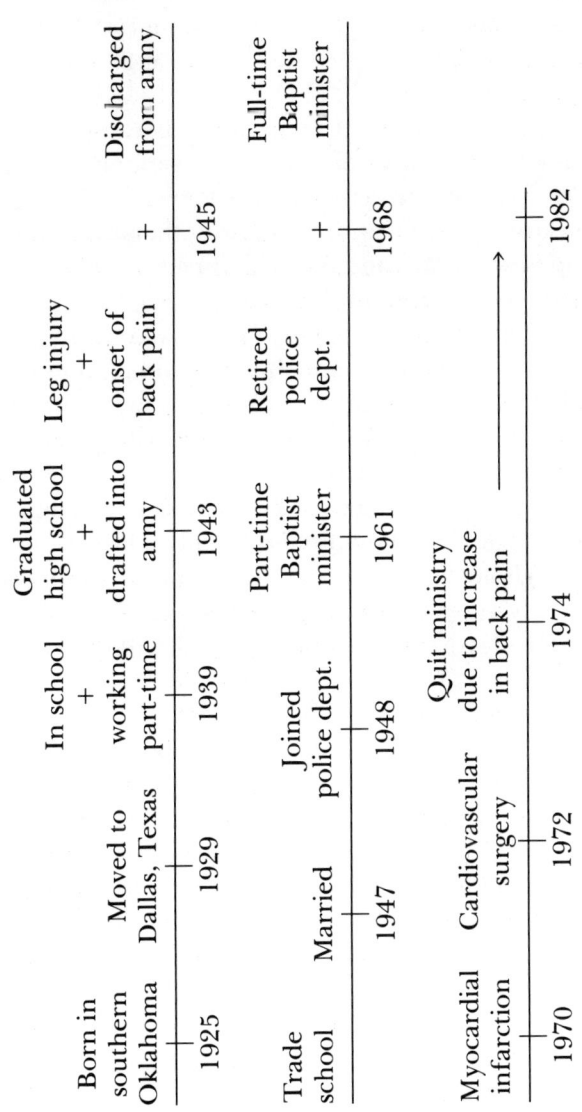

Figure 5.1   *Chronology of significant events in the life of John Calvin Smithson*

Soon after graduation, John was drafted into the army. He spent 28 months in the army, 14 of which were in combat situations during World War II. Early in military life, John contracted dysentery for 90 days and lost between fifty and sixty pounds. Thereafter, he was transferred and contracted malaria. After recovering from malaria, he was sent into combat. John spent some 150 days in 24-hour combat. During the last 2 to 3 weeks of combat he was wounded in his left thigh.

In John's estimation, the wound occurred because "an idiot from quartermaster became my company commander." He described this major as untrained in combat, yet having a "big ego like all those other damn officers." John and two others were sent up to a mountaintop to see if "anyone shoots at them," despite his attempts to explain that the mountaintop was a "zeroing range for artillery every night." The major sent them up anyway to dig in for the night, "so I went." After he and his two companions dug in, it became dark and the shelling started, lasting two hours. Once the shelling ended, John's buddy lit a match and "saw the enemy crawling all over the place." John stated, "you better start shooting." John related that his companion in the next foxhole stood up, got his ear shot off, and fled down the mountain. Enemy soldiers took over the abandoned foxhole and John "was in hand-to-hand combat all night." He used up one case of grenades and exhausted his rifle ammunition. At daybreak, the enemy had disappeared.

During the night, John had received a flesh wound to his left thigh from a bullet. The bullet had not struck the bone but "severed all my nerves in my leg cause it has been weak and numb since; I still have severe pain in my leg." As John headed down the mountain that day, he used two rifles as crutches. During his descent, a sniper with a machine gun fired at John and he "tumbled about 100–150 yards down." When he recovered, he had "pain all over . . . particularly in my back." John stated that during this time period he had not bathed nor changed his socks nor brushed his teeth for six months, and "was in terrible shape, but them idiots wanted to send me back into combat." Instead, John left on his own to the battalion first-aid station and demanded to see a physician. The physician reclassified him as "unfit for duty" and sent him home. He was able to obtain a discharge from the army because he had "accumulated enough points for discharge." He then spent the next several months recuperating in various military hospitals outside the United States.

John described the general conditions of combat as horrible. He had spent an extended period of time in combat. He reported that for six months he had been in combat during the rainy season. During one period, it had rained for fourteen straight days and nights; and he had spent each night sleeping in water. After this period, John could not walk for two months due to "jungle rot" of his feet. His teeth had rotted and he lost them.

After his flesh wound to his left thigh, he was reclassified as noncombat and was discharged several months later. John was twenty years old at the time of discharge. He was discharged in Arkansas and urged to go into the Veterans Administration hospital for full recovery from his various physical and "nervous" conditions. John declined and went home to Texas, because he was homesick. He now states, "that's where I made my mistake" by not going into the VA hospital. At discharge, he had received 60 percent disability due to his wounds, jungle rot, nerves, and malaria. Over a two-year period, the disability was halved to 30 percent and it was increased to 100 percent in 1978. John spent thirty days after his discharge just "trying to eat well and regain my weight."

After being discharged for one year, John married in 1947 and has been married for thirty-six years. After being discharged, he could not obtain a job and decided to go to a plumbing training program for nine months. The VA paid his tuition. After completing this program, the only job he could find was a part-time position. A friend told him about openings in the Dallas police department. John applied and was accepted. John's father and uncle had been police officers and that somewhat influenced his decision to join.

John performed three different roles as a police officer. The first three years were spent in a "scout car," which is a patrol car. John related that while on patrol-car duty for three years, he never experienced a life-threatening situation. His biggest problems were "his bosses." They were "idiots." One in particular "was one of those hard-nosed young ones with no experience." After getting off duty one night, John was sitting down filling out forms and "this turkey came up to me and started cussing me and I hadn't said a word, . . . I just got up and walked out. . . . He done a lot of people that way. . . . When I was on graveyard shift, that turkey would follow us all night long for no reason." One night, however, John turned the tables. The supervisor was following John one evening in a vehicle with its lights turned off. John "whipped" around a corner behind a grocery store. The supervisor was sitting in the middle of the intersection with his lights out looking for him. John stated "I pulled up behind him and rammed his rear" at twenty miles per hour. John then walked up to the supervisor and said, "'I didn't see you there with your lights out,' and [the supervisor] was white as a sheet, and he didn't follow me anymore."

After patrol-car duty, John volunteered for motorcycle duty. He wanted motorcycle duty because there was no radio installed on the vehicles, and he felt he could thus be "his own boss." John stayed on motorcycle duty for twelve years, then spent five years in the warrant office. He served traffic and criminal warrants. The most memorable incident John recalled had occurred while he was serving warrants. One schoolteacher had $600 worth of traffic tickets, and John went to her home to serve a warrant. "She offered me a drink and turned sweet to me." John recognized her as one of his son's English teachers. He told her, "Jack is my son, and you flunked him in English." Next semester, John reports that Jack got an *A* in English.

John retired from the police department in 1968, after putting in twenty years. He retired because "it was too much of a strain . . . a rat race," and "the supervisors made it bad."

During the last seven years of John's employment with the police force, he had become a part-time minister with a Baptist church. He had been going to church all his life and was devoted to his religion. He felt an urge to "preach his experience and thoughts," because he considered himself a moral person. After retiring from the police force, John became a full-time minister for six years. He stated that being a "pastor was worse than being in a police department cause there was too many nuts to deal with."

During those thirteen years, John's back and leg pain became worse; and he retired from the church in 1974. He stated that the "two most strenuous occupations as far as physical and mental strain is being a police officer and a minister . . . that's a fact!" John stated that more ministers than any other profession die of heart attacks due to stress. John himself had sustained a heart attack in 1970. He stated that stress was always a problem, because "you done what you know is right and have the proper motives; and everytime you do it, they [the congregation] pull the rug out from under you." Although he did not wish to further elaborate on these difficulties, he finally quit the church in 1974 due to his chronic, daily back pains.

John considered his marriage to be a good one. He has three grown children: two sons and one daughter. Both sons have families. The daughter is single and manages a clothing store. John does not smoke or drink. The last eight years have been spent mainly in bed due to his back condition.

MEDICAL HISTORY OF JOHN CALVIN SMITHSON

John's current major medical problem is "severe degenerative disc disease secondary to severe osteoarthritis" (obtained from his medical record at the VA). John relates the origin of this to his leg injury in World War II. The bullet wound shortened his left leg, which "twisted my back" and later "my disc ruptured" due to the twisted back. Since 1974, John reports suffering from chronic, twenty-four-hour pain in his lower back. John had suffered back pain since he was injured in World War II, but states "I could live with it and it didn't stop me from working. . . . It got progressive and in seventy-four, I had to quit." He indicates that since 1974, "sometimes it would pinch nerves in sciatic nerves . . . off and on . . . and when it does . . . I have to stay in bed."

Prior to 1974, John did not go to the VA for his back. He went to several doctors in the Dallas area. The first doctors he saw were doctors whom the city (police department) sent him to. The first doctor "was getting paid off not to find anything since it was close to retirement." A mylogram was performed that turned out to be negative, and John suffered from headaches for thirty days due to the mylogram. The first doctor did not find anything wrong, so John complained and was sent to another doctor. The second doctor also told John that nothing could be found wrong with his back.

Once John started going to the back clinic at the VA, he was told he had osteoarthritis. He has tried every treatment presented to him by the VA with little success. Treatments included analgesics, anti-inflammatory agents, exercise, braces, biofeedback, and transcutaneous nerve stimulation. John has been provided with braces, back corsets, two wheelchairs, a french cane, a whirlpool, transcutaneous nerve stimulators, and medicines from the VA.

Sine 1974, John has not only been treated by the VA, but has sought out other remedies with his own funds. He has seen three different chiropractors ("only one has helped"), an acupuncturist, and various orthopedic specialists and generalists. The VA in Dallas sent him to a back specialist in the Houston VA, and the doctor told John: "I wouldn't touch your back with a thirty-foot pole." By John's account, he has been victimized by several physicians. One gave him "hormone shots" at fifty dollars a shot, and the shots made him worse. Six months ago, the VA sent John to an arthritis clinic in Houston, Texas. John said: "People go there from all over the world." The doctors at the clinic put him on calcium. They also put him on antidepressant medication, but John had to stop using it because antidepressants made him more depressed.

Due to John's medical condition, he is 100 percent disabled. For the last four to five years, he has only been able to sit up for a period of one to three hours a day due to back pain. His home has been modified to suit his disability. Figure 5.2 is a sketch of John's home. He has two personal bedrooms. One contains a hospital bed and mattress, and the other contains a waterbed. The waterbed "helps more than anything else I've tried." A whirlpool is connected to his bathtub in the bathroom. The living-den area has been expanded, and the walls have been designed to let in much sunlight, i.e., more and larger windows. Another reason for modification is to have the dining area in this large room. This allows John easier accessibility. John is ambulatory only to go to the bathroom when he can. In other words, if the pain is not too severe, he can walk to the bathroom; if the pain is too severe, he has a urinal and bedpan at his bedside. Through a typical twenty-four-hour day in the last four to six years, John spends one to three hours in a recliner, about twenty hours in bed and one to two hours in the bathtub. The VA was going to build a concrete runway to his front door to make it accessible by wheelchair, but John thought "they would screw it up." To make entering the house easier, John had sliding glass doors installed in the large expanded room at ground level, so he can be wheelchaired in through the rear entrance directly from a car.

John's back disability has affected his wife. For many years, she did not "fully" believe the extent of his disability, because she has some arthritis also. She is very supportive, however, and her life revolves around John. She has learned recently how to cope with his pain. She describes her life as "a twenty-four-hour private nurse," but accepts it because she loves her husband. She believes the VA has offered John all they can offer; therefore, she is not hostile toward the VA.

One of John's daughters-in-law, along with her three girls, is not allowed to visit John's home any longer. John talks about the girls "not minding and always fighting." He can't stand the noise and disobedience. When they came in, his back pain would get worse, and John would have to retreat to the bedroom and close the door. John had discussed this with his daughter-in-law several times, but nothing changed; therefore he does not allow them in his house at this time. John's wife does not totally agree with her husband but "respects" his decision.

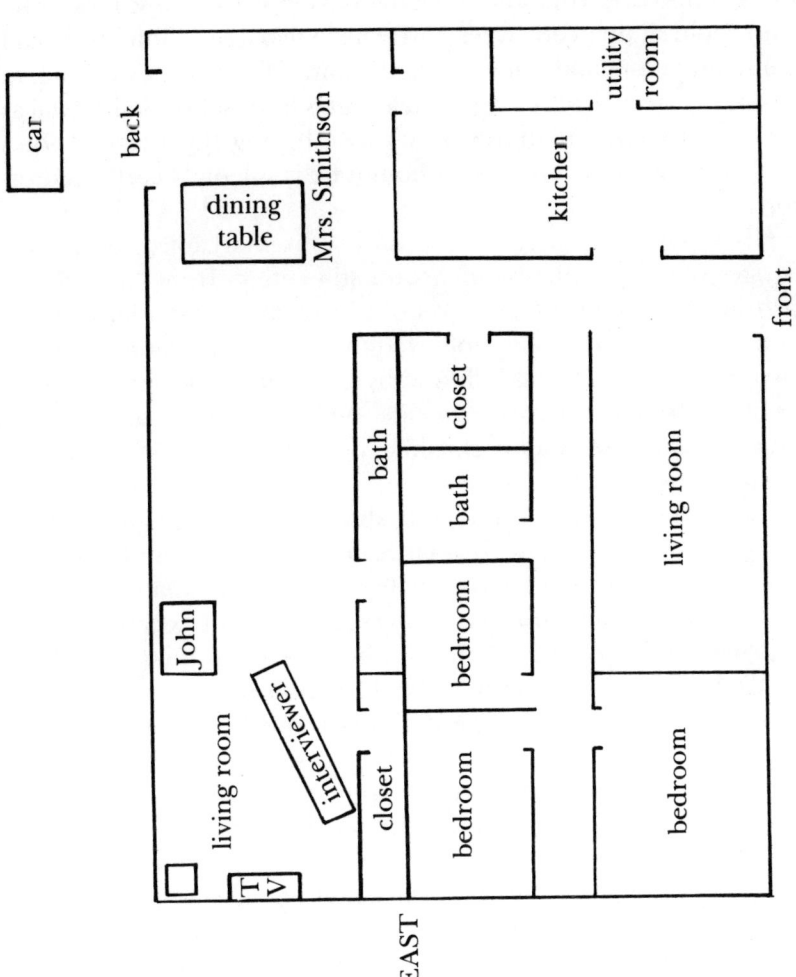

Figure 5.2   Floor plan of John Smithson's home

John's other major medical problem involves his heart. He had a heart attack in 1970 and "was dead three times in the ambulance." He was hospitalized for twenty-eight days and stayed in bed at home for thirty more days. John had a friend in a produce stand who brought him raw fruits and vegetables. After eating these foods raw, John could sit up in one week and walk in two weeks. John had read about nutrition and thus "healed" himself. In 1972, John had coronary-artery bypass surgery at a Dallas Baptist hospital as well as a left ventricular aneurysectomy. Since having this surgery, John has had no heart symptoms, although he is still on "heart" medications.

His other medical history is fairly unremarkable, i.e., a cholecystectomy and pneumonia. John still suffers from "jungle rot" rash in the summer. He breaks out in pustules, especially on his feet. He is currently being followed in the VA's dermatology clinic. Currently, John is being followed by three different physicians for his back condition. Two are outside the VA system. In addition, he visits regularly the VA's back clinic, dermatology clinic, eye clinic, and arthritis clinic.

John has two major complaints about the VA and "government medicine." One deals with holistic medicine. He thinks the VA should get involved in holistic medicine, for he has read a lot about it. His other major complaint involves lack of use of experimental or unproven drugs by the VA. John uses dimethyl sulfoxide (DMSO) for his back, and it works well for three hours as an analgesic. He does not use it often because it stinks. His concoction consists of a 30 percent DMSO and 70 percent grain-alcohol mixture that "settles" for two to three days before he applies it. John talked about a venom from a red ant in South America that cures anything, and "I know our government has it . . . because I've read about it in Washington newspapers." He feels the same about laetrile and other drugs being used in European countries. He can't understand why more is not being done to develop these drugs for use in the United States.

Interview Case Summary

The interviews with John Calvin Smithson took place in his home. Mr. Smithson was sitting up in his lounge chair, which faces east. The interviewer sat north of him on the couch, and Mrs. Smithson sat behind the interviewer. At first the interviewer felt somewhat uncomfortable having one person in front of him and one behind. Mrs. Smithson tended to be protective of her husband.

She went quickly to his side to get him something or to answer the phone, and she seemed to "rush" when he needed something.

John C. Smithson is an interesting and intelligent person. He is very knowledgeable about the medical field in general. John related the genesis of his back pain to an injury in World War II, when he was only nineteen or twenty years old. Whether or not he suffered from back pain for fifteen to twenty years before getting VA help cannot be answered with certainty from these interviews. To be specific, he did not seek help until his retirement year from the police force in 1968. By his own account however, John's history of back pain started before his army discharge. His presentation of back problems during the interviews was sketchy and questionable to the interviewer. He had been able to run, jump, etc.; and he had been required to pass physicals in order to be a police officer. John simply stated that he had learned to live with some degree of pain, and the pain had become progressively more intense as time went by and occurred more frequently. He does not recall any injuries to his back or legs since the injury in World War II.

There is no doubt that Mr. Smithson has severe osteoarthritis with severe degenerative disc disease in his lower back. He states unwillingness to accept additional "standard" therapies that have been presented to him, until someone can present the new "experimental" drugs that he mentioned. When the interviewer had first arrived at his home, his wife was applying peanut oil to his back, as Mr. Smithson had just read that it can cure arthritis.

Mr. Smithson's life, past and present, revolves around his back pain. He is set in his daily routines. He states that he currently visits the VA infrequently as a result of waiting time to see a doctor and prolonged recovery time to "get over" the trips to the clinics. Mr. Smithson feels that he should be seen immediately when he goes to a clinic, because he is a "bed patient." He had to sit for three hours to be seen on his last visit. It takes him two weeks of bedrest to recover from one trip to the VA. He complains of suffering twenty-four hours a day.

John's providers at the VA have used all their resources in trying to ease his pain and help him cope with his situation. Personnel in physical therapy and rehabilitation don't remember Mr. Smithson specifically, however, as "we have so many like him" to deal with.

The interviewer talked with the "outcast" daughter-in-law and her husband. She stated feeling that her father-in-law is "cold and self-serving" and that she doesn't understand him. She is anxious to follow his wishes about not visiting him. His son tries to help him in any way that he can. He feels that his father has taught him a lot, and he will always support him. His son plans to build him a sundeck on top of the carport this summer, so he can enjoy the summer sun's pleasant warmth on his back. The interviewer was uncertain how Mr. Smithson was to climb one flight of stairs, or reach the carport roof.

In the interviewer's estimation, John had portrayed a "defeatist" attitude. John's "pain" had won the war but maybe not the battle, as he hoped for new treatments and drugs. Throughout the interviews, Mr. Smithson's attitude was reflected in his views of social and political events. For example, John believed that Nelson Rockefeller controlled the world's wealth with his position in the "Trilateral Commission." The interviewer recommended that Mr. Smithson receive some type of psychiatric counseling away from the VA or any government facility. He concluded from his interviews that Mr. Smithson needs someone competent to discuss with him the pros and cons of experimental drugs or venoms. He recommended family counseling as well.

COMMENTARY (Stein)

Mr. Roediger's descriptive study amply documents what we all—even if only intuitively—know to be a fact: that a human life has but a single history. In it interweave what *we* have compartmentalized into (1) medical history, (2) occupational history, (3) family history, and so on. All these histories are *cultural* compartmentalizations based upon a selection of certain *types* of information that reflect our interest as investigators or clinicians. Still, these various histories are our *organizations* of reality, not reality itself. To restrict our field of inquiry by selecting out certain variables (i.e., types of data) to study is legitimate only insofar as we also recognize that such divisions are artificial and *might* exclude precisely what we need in order to explain and intervene. Neither disease nor treatment exists in a vacuum. We need to know what *contexts* produce, nourish, sustain, or diminish the disease. We need to know the meaning of illness in the lives of the patient, family, and health care providers alike.

Mr. Smithson's health actions offer us some clue as to the "health belief model" (see Jette et al. 1981) according to which he operates. He has long relied on the official governmental (VA) and biomedical system as his place of first resort. As this repeatedly fails him, he has sought cure from such alternate health care approaches as chiropractic, DMSO therapy, and rubdowns of peanut oil administered by his wife. It must be noted that he expects complete cure, and therefore pursues it through literature and fantasy (I am here specifically thinking of his fantasy that Nelson Rockefeller and the Trilateral Commission ultimately controls his access to cure).

A number of conspicuous themes in the life of John Calvin Smithson can be identified: (1) the litany of unfair bosses, (2) his feeling of unending victimization at the hands of others who are stupid or capricious, (3) his allocation to others of all responsibility for and control over his life, (4) his conflict between wishing to take control over his own life and his dependency upon and resentment of others, (5) his need to be policeman and moral "policeman" (minister), versus his inability to "police" himself, (6) his use of pain to punish himself and others (and likewise to control them), (7) his use of pain to express his grievance against the world, together with (8) his quasi-paranoid conviction that there is help (cure, salvation) out there somewhere, but that person(s) in power is (are) withholding it from him. The problematic character of his manliness (gender identity) haunts all his multiple histories and life themes.

It would be a grievous error to take John at his word with respect to the debilitating nature of his pain, for he is not so much unemployed as "pain" has become his full-time occupation. Seen this way, he employs countless others, in his family and in medicine, to work for and under him. His pain enables him to be boss and to get away with it. Thus, the sequence soldier, policeman, minister, pain patient is *continuous* rather than discontinuous.

Mr. Smithson has a deep grievance against life: medical treatment is payment in part for a debt that can never be fully repaid. His use of pain and disability as a passive-dependent, but also passive-aggressive, form of *revenge* can be seen more clearly if we juxtapose against this case the opening soliloquy of Shakespeare's *King Richard the Third*. Richard, Duke of Gloucester, seeks to set his brother George, Duke of Clarence, against their brother King Edward IV. With distilled "narcissistic rage" (Kohut 1972), he filters his envy to the undoing of the entire royal house:

> *Now is the winter of our discontent*
> *Made glorious summer by this sun of York;*
> *And all the clouds that lour'd upon our house*
> *In the deep bosom of the ocean buried.*
> *Now are our brows bound with victorious wreaths;*
> *Our bruised arms hung up for monuments;*
> *Our stern alarums chang'd to merry meetings,*

Our dreadful marches to delightful measures.
Grim-visag'd war hath smooth'd his wrinkled front,
And now, instead of mounting barbed steeds
To fright the souls of fearful adversaries,
He capers nimbly in a lady's chamber
To the lascivious pleasing of a lute.
But I—that am not shap'd for sportive tricks,
Nor made to court an amorous looking-glass—
I—that am rudely stamp'd, and want love's majesty
To strut before a wanton ambling nymph—
I—that am curtail'd of this fair proportion,
Cheated of feature by dissembling nature,
Deform'd, unfinish'd, sent before my time
Into this breathing world scarce half made up,
And that so lamely and unfashionable
That dogs bark at me as I halt by them—
Why, I, in this weak piping time of peace,
Have no delight to pass away the time,
Unless to spy my shadow in the sun
And descant on mine own deformity.
And therefore, since I cannot prove a lover
To entertain these fair well-spoken days,
I am determined to prove a villain
And hate the idle pleasures of these days.
Plots have I laid, inductions dangerous.
By drunken prophecies, libels, and dreams,
To set my brother Clarence and the King
In deadly hate the one against the other;
And if King Edward be as true and just
As I am subtle, false, and treacherous,
This day should Clarence closely be mew'd up—
About a prophecy which says that G
of Edward's heirs the murderer shall be.
Dive, thoughts, down to my soul. Here Clarence comes.

(Alexander 1952:701–2).

Far more is at work in this case than simple iatrogenesis: indeed, iatrogenesis is more often than not a rhetorical epithet applied from the outside to affix blame and to absolve oneself. If there is iatrogenesis here, then it involves more than cause and effect. Iatrogenesis here has more the character of *complicity* than anything else. It would be more accurate, from a "systems" point of view, to say that where medicine went wrong was in trying too hard to help the patient by complying with his demand for treatment. Over the patient's long medical history, one sees a mutual "complementary" (Bateson 1972) escalation whereby the more care that is provided (analgesics, braces, biofeedback, nerve stimulators, wheelchairs . . .) the more John Calvin Smithson regresses. The more his family and health-care providers overfunction, the more he underfunctions—to the point of invalidism (Bowen 1978). The more medicine tries to be the good parent, the more the patient becomes the bad child. He can hardly be expected to comply with medicine in rehabilitating himself when medicine tacitly and unwittingly complies with his wish not to be rehabilitated. His "life-style" of illness is not simply a personal maladaptation: it is a *mutual* maladaptation between patient, family, medicine, and the wider society. Over the years, we have often branded him as a malingerer. Yet his largely subjective pain is nonetheless real. It is not feigned. *Malingerer* describes how we *feel* about the patient in the guise of attributes that we have attributed to him (e.g., willful defiance, faking, etc.). It is moral condemnation in the language of clinical judgment.

His life themes, outlined above, could well predict the vicissitudes of his illness. His "representational world" (that inner unconscious template that gives form and meaning to experience, Stolorow and Atwood 1979:43) is peopled by illegitimate male authorities who collectively are "stupid" and "idiots"; it is one in which others have consistently let him down and owe him a debt that they can never repay, yet that he persistently tries to exact; one in which anything unpleasant that happens to him is always someone else's fault. Yet he could not succeed in becoming a male authority in his own right. His repeated failures at *policing others*, together with his consistent *inability to police himself*, suggests that his life course has been one of persistent decompensation and socially acceptable defenses (soldier, patrol and motorcycle policeman, minister, finally unrepentant patient!) that work temporarily. He is a policeman who accepts bribes. He hates the law he cannot uphold. Perhaps etymology can assist us: his *pain* is his *penalty*, his *punishment*. (The medical, legal, and religious are different *institutions* that share the same overarching *ethos*). To a considerable extent, he has now allocated superego or conscience functions to others, just as— successfully only for a while—he tried to be an external policeman for others. His reaction formations and undoing were undermined by a return of the repressed; as a result, his current *solution* (in the guise of the sick role as a problem for *others* to solve) is to punish others and himself by being condemned to the sick role. He stead-fastly believes that the "goodness" that could cure him exists *outside himself,* but that somebody "out there" is pulling the strings to withhold his redemption, to deprive him of health. His life history comes to look like an endless pilgrimage, ever unfulfilled. Today he seeks a miraculously achieved pain-free life. Medicine is now his failed religion. Every salvation eludes his failing grasp. A lifelong seeker of redemption from suffering, he is condemned to suffer.

What others call his manipulation corresponds to their need to care and help. Medicine must try to cure: it both *must* help and *cannot* help because, in the patient's scheme of things, nobody is ever good enough. As he says, life is always "pulling the rug out from under you." Still, *his* meanings subvert medicine's best inten-tions: psychologically, he pulls the rug out from beneath medicine. He cannot be cured not only for medical reasons but for psychologi-cal ones as well.

Midwestern, highly Baptist-influenced sex-role expectations help us to understand the patient's ambivalence over dependency and his management of aggression (Stein 1987). A male must strive to demonstrate his independence while craving the tenderness he must renounce. Century-old cowboy ballads and contemporary country-and-western songs attest to the persistence of this theme. A "real man" would never admit to wanting to be taken care of. Acceptance of the sick role as *permanent* status is tantamount to electing to be symbolically castrated, feminized—which in turn leads him to insist that he does not *wish* to be dependent. His regression both fulfills a forbidden wish and unleashes a protest masculinity that repudiates the wish. Moreover, all semblance of aggression must be eradicated, for Baptists pride themselves on their virtual inability to be angry. Not only must one not show his anger to another, he must not feel that forbidden part to be present in himself. As one recent Baptist church billboard read: "Anger is but one letter away from danger." The patient's aggression becomes acceptably expressed through disingenuous smiles, self-effacing humor, passive-aggressive behavior, and projection (whereby anger and malice are attributed to others). The price of love is the disown-ing of anger: therefore, to show any direct anger to his family or health caretakers would be to court the danger of losing them. Yet it is equally intolerable to put oneself at the mercy of others' unreliable intentions. The cowboy wishes only to have his comforting solitude.

Seen from the outside, or from the frustration of family and health care personnel, the patient's pain rules everyone's behavior.

Yet seen from within the system, he neither causes nor especially dominates others' behavior so much as they share a common set of rules. One could just as well argue that he complies with others' rules! What, indeed, would they *all* do without each other, and without his symptoms? What, one must ask, are they *not* attending to that is conveniently and consensually displaced onto him and his full-time care? How then could he be rehabilitated if somehow his condition is necessary to the psychic functioning of the family and the wider system? Seen thus, his problems are in fact implicit *solutions*.

While Smithson's demands for ever more regressively infantile status have been met by his ever-widening network of caretakers, those very demands reflect an unconscious setting of rules by those around him to which he is conscientiously adhering. Stated differently, noncompliance is a tacit form of compliance, for caretakers and patient are in fact complying with one another. In a symmetrical spiral that has the armaments race as analogue, the greater the patient's dependency needs, the greater is the environment's effort to meet them (expecting clinical success from so doing); and conversely, the more his environment tries to help, the more petulantly dependent he becomes.

Patient and cadre of healers, of course, profoundly resent one another, a resentment that surfaces in outbursts of indirection, as each escalates the passive-aggressive warfare from which there is no extrication. Health care personnel, at the end of their rope, will resort to triage and turfing (that is, refer the patient to yet another service, whereupon the old cycle recommences). For his part, Mr. Smithson becomes frustrated with his treatment, abandons it for yet some other miraculous medical whim he has discovered, only to find rejection and disappointment anew. What is ostensibly a caretaking relationship subtly and quickly becomes a mutually punitive, sadomasochistic one.

Cost-effectiveness, hospital utilization, and other issues related to reality testing all become shipwrecked by unconscious issues that lurk beneath the surface. Where generalized intervention has itself become the problem (which takes us now into the arena of public policy), how can we expect more intervention to be the remedy except in a magical way? Is Mr. Smithson alone to be faulted if family, health care personnel, medical institutions, government policymakers, and finally the electorate have themselves abandoned the search for maturity and have set in its place the illusion of unlimited collective breasts available for infinite oral incorporation?

Stated differently, why should Mr. Smithson relinquish the satisfactions of infantile dependency for the vicissitudes of autonomy, responsibility, and maturity when his caretakers tenaciously adhere to him to avoid their own autonomy, responsibility, and maturity?[1]

The cumulative effect of the case is that of sheer exhaustion, defeat, futility. The patient "makes" us feel that we are dealing with a defiantly bad boy who not only will not improve or comply but who refuses to be grateful for all our collective efforts. He brings out the wish to punish him; but, guilty from the very thought, we try even harder to help. His increased helplessness induces in his caretakers an even more despairing sense of helplessness (and their sense of failure evokes his deepened dependency); as his care givers feel that they are failing him, they widen the circle of care by accumulating consultations with yet other experts who might help them to help him. Everyone in the system comes to feel inadequate and blames others within the system for the sad turn of events. To put it another way, the system is sustained on reciprocal projection. What is even worse, now that Mr. Smithson's considerable muscular atrophy (presumably irreversible) has taken place, it appears that the system now faces a collectively created "self-fulfilling prophecy."

In the face of the patient's history and previous health-care efforts, what dare one audaciously recommend? Put another way: What kinds of solutions would not simply feed into and perpetuate the very problem they are designed to solve?

(1) Less is more. His anxiety induces anxiety in his care givers to continue to try to *do something*. Often the very "doing" is an attempt by the care givers to assuage their own anxiety and guilt. One can help him, his family, and other patients like him by containing rather than expanding the problem.

(2) Acknowledge, through an understanding of one's own *counter-transference* (see Stein 1982b, 1983, 1985), the patient's rage, feelings of inadequacy, despair, emasculation, etc. The patient wishes not to feel these things either, but to project them into health care personnel and family members so that they will feel compelled to take these feelings away (a magical, and realistically impossible wish).

(3) Help the patient find even miniscule areas in his life in which he can feel competent and responsible, and therefore more of a man. He would then feel more in control of himself, and feel less

---

[1] In my formulation of this paragraph, I am endebted to Professor Arthur E. Hippler, who generously commented on an earlier version of this essay (23 March 1983).

driven to control others in his behalf. Everyone in the system has colluded with his definition that disease is his life. But there is more to him than his afflictions. Yet no one has taken an interest in him, and in his possible contributions to others, apart from his pathologies and debilities.

(4) Help his wife and other family members to take a few individuating steps for themselves. Their entire lives are built around him in an effort to do penance for their real and imagined wrongdoings and guilts. In helping them to draw boundaries around themselves, one indirectly helps him to differentiate a self less intruded upon by others whom he so desperately draws to him *and* repels.

(5) Finally, as this entire case has suggested, one must learn to take more cues from the context and not simply from the disease process, since the latter does not exist in a social vacuum. Closer attention to this context will provide the suggestions as to how and how not to intervene in the future.

REFERENCES

Alexander, P., ed. 1952. King Richard the Third, act 1, scene 1. In *William Shakespeare: The complete works,* 701–2. New York: Random House.

Bateson, G. 1972. *Steps to an ecology of mind: Collected essays in anthropology, psychiatry, evolution, and epistemology.* San Francisco: Chandler.

Bowen, M. 1978. *Family therapy in clinical practice.* New York: Jason Aronson.

Eisenberg, L., and A. Kleinman, eds. 1981. *The relevance of social science for medicine.* Boston: D. Reidel.

Jette, A. M., K. M. Cummings, B. M. Brock, M. C. Phelps, and J. Naessens. 1981. The structure and reliability of health belief indices. *Health Services Research* 16(1):81–98.

Kleinman, A. 1980. *Patients and healers in the context of culture: An exploration of the borderland between anthropology, medicine, and psychiatry.* Berkeley and Los Angeles: University of California Press.

Kohut, H. 1972. Thoughts on narcissism and narcissistic rage. *The psychoanalytic study of the child* 27:360–400. New York: Quadrangle/The New York Times Press.

Stein, H. F. 1980. Review essay on *Patients and healers in the context of culture,* by A. Kleinman. *The Journal of Psychological Anthropology* 3(2):197–204.

———. 1982a. The contest for control: A case of diabetes mellitus in psychosomatic, familial health care, and cultural contexts. *The Journal of Psychoanalytic Anthropology* 5(2):173–96.

———. 1982b. Physician-patient transaction through the analysis of countertransference: A study in role relationship and unconscious meaning. *Medical Anthropology* 6(3):165–82.

———. 1983. The influence of counter-transference upon the clinical relationship and decision-making. *Continuing Education for the Family Physician* 18(7):625–30.

————. 1985. Whatever happened to counter-transference? The subjective in medicine. In *Context and dynamics in clinical knowledge*, vol. 1 of the Series in Ethnicity, Medicine, and Psychoanalysis, by H. F. Stein, and M. Apprey, 1–55. Charlottesville: University Press of Virginia.

————. 1987. Farmer and cowboy: The duality of the Midwestern male ethos—A study in ethnicity, regionalism, and national identity. In *From metaphor to meaning: Papers in psychoanalytic anthropology*, vol. 2 of the Series in Ethnicity, Medicine, and Psychoanalysis, by H. F. Stein, and M. Apprey, 178–227. Charlottesville: University Press of Virginia.

Stolorow, R. D., and G. E. Atwood. 1979. *Faces in a cloud.* New York: Aronson.

PART II

Stories and
Their Translations in
Clinical Education
and Supervision

CHAPTER 6

Bridging the Gap via Context: An Ethnographic Clinical-Training Model

HOWARD F. STEIN

PROLOGUE

A generation or so ago, before I was properly trained, I was deeply affected by Paul Tillich's *The Courage to Be* and *The Shaking of the Foundations*, Bishop John A. T. Robinson's *Honest to God*, and Martin Buber's *I and Thou* and *Between Man and Man,* works that all strived to penetrate or transcend—depending on your metaphor—the institutional metaphysical, doctrinal, and mythological architecture of Western religions in order to find what was true and basic about life. Now, properly trained and credentialed as a medical anthropologist and clinical teacher, I adamantly refuse to relinquish or renounce my earlier heresy. Indeed, I discover that I have merely transposed the message of these earlier works into a new and different key, from the idiom of religion to that of medicine and science. I still refuse to believe that truth, wisdom, and other ultimate concerns are to be discovered by aligning myself with doctrinal orthodoxy or are measurable in terms of institutional loyalties.

Although I shall diligently try to offer you an intellectually compelling and clinically plausible model for bridging the gap or chasm between biomedicine and the behavioral sciences, and shall even boast of a modicum of success for having spanned the disciplinary Dardanelles myself, I want you to know from the outset that deep down, I know—and I know that you know—that both sides or poles of this forbidding gap are our cherished illusions, figments of our collective and historical imagination, our words become printed flesh. I do not "believe in" either side of the Straits. When we choose sides, we defend our respective side of the abyss as if our very identities depended on it, as if a viewpoint were reality itself. Certainly, in academic disciplines we do not go so far as to kill for the sake of these group identities—that, at least, is only done in the name of religion, nation, ethnicity, and politics. Ultimately, I am less interested in merely bridging the gap than in understanding why human beings everywhere create such gaps between "us" and "them" (Stein 1985d, 1987a; GAP Committee on International Relations and Stein 1987), gaps that we then try ecumenically— often feigning more than honestly grappling—to bridge. I trust my heresy; it is my conceptual framework, my modus operandi, and my faith. I believe, with Martin Buber, that truth—including clinical truth—lies "between." The issue is not, or at least should not be, bridging disciplines A and B, but teaching patient care. That deserves to be the unshakable foundation of all that we do.

INTRODUCTION

This chapter is an example of psychoanalytically informed, and systems-thinking-deepened, applied anthropology. It represents an effort to integrate a number of social and behavioral sciences (anthropology, psychoanalysis, family systems, cybernetics, psychohistory, small-group theory, political psychology) in clinical teaching together with the biomedical specialty of family medicine. It would be simplistic and wrongheaded for me to say that it represents an attempt to bridge the gap between behavioral sciences and family medicine, as if either of the two were monoliths. Intellectual and clinical engineers that we are, we know that we have our hands plenty full to build countless bridges over many troubled contexts. Many chasms have yet to be bridged, including between the numerous feuding behavioral sciences as well as between the biomedical specialties, each devising corporate raids upon the others. If we permit ourselves to think of professional societies and of academic disciplines as bona fide *cultures,* then we might say that this chapter is an exercise in multicultural and intercultural communication— and a portrait of limits set upon it.

Let me begin by offering a few definitions. *Ethnography* refers to the detailed description and interpretation of a group's way of life, its beliefs, values, expectations, rules, conscious and unconscious levels of meaning, attitudes, roles, and the consequences of all these for behavior. One strives to learn how the "natives" see, feel, experience their world, what from linguistics is called the "emic" viewpoint (i.e., the farmer who plows Mother Earth versus the farmer who plows a fall acreage of financial investment). While this cultural

construction of reality often differs markedly from that of the observer—this latter called "etic," again from linguistics—one goal of
ethnographic work is to help build a corpus of comparative cross-
cultural studies that further permit one to develop a comprehensive
ethnological theory, not only about that individual group, but about
commonalities and variations in being human. Ideally, these methods and models help us to know what is culture- or era-specific, and
what is species-specific, that is, universal. Now, given our Babel of
claims to being uniquely scientific (science's version of ethnocen-
trism!), in the dialogue between family medicine and family therapy, or for that matter, between family systems thinking and sociology, the question as to which is the "emic" and which the "etic"
reduces to "Who is looking askance at whom?" Sciences—like ethnic groups, nations, and religions—experience what George De Vos
(1966) called "status anxiety" as they compare themselves with
others, hoping to be superior.

At any rate, the ethnographic method—which can be dated from
the anthropological work of Bronislaw Malinowski in the Trobriand
Islands, off northern Papua New Guinea during the First World
War—is the process of systematically eliciting knowledge of what it
is like to live as a member of a particular group. Methods or techniques commonly used in ethnographic research are naturalistic
and participant observation; open-ended or nondirective interview; long-term, intimate familiarity with the group by working
closely, if not living, with them, often for years; and the selection
of a number of key "informants," people knowledgeable of the
group's meanings and history, to help one navigate, expand one's
network, and avoid getting into too much trouble (taboo toxicities).
This all becomes "applied" in addition to "theoretical" anthropology, when the goal is to *help the group studied to do something* (e.g.,
change) rather than simply to use knowledge derived from the
study to build theory (and careers in more academic anthropology
departments). Any self-respecting anthropologist who reads this
collapse of a near century of research into a page and a half will
surely bristle in disbelief at the distortions I have allowed. However,
since the point of this chapter is that everything is contextual,
including this very chapter, I am satisfied to end the truncated
history lesson here.

In their classic, *Pragmatics of Human Communication,* Watzlawick,
Beavin, and Jackson wrote (1967:20–21) that "[A] phenomenon
remains unexplainable as long as the range of observations is not
wide enough to include the context in which the phenomenon

occurs." While this elegant formulation is true, to be more true one must add to the *range* or *breadth* of observations their *depth* as well. Observational and clinical contexts are not only composed of assorted personnel and social *units*—individuals, families, institutions, communities, cultures—in various *relationships;* but in addition these units and relationships are themselves *unconsciously linked* by out-of-awareness feelings, meanings, fantasies, and wishes. In my clinical teaching and theoretical work, I have been striving to build what might be called a *psychoanalytic systems theory* (Stein 1982a, 1985a, 1985c; Stein and Apprey 1985, 1987)—a phrase that to some might be a heresy and to others an oxymoron!

As if this contextual complexity were not overwhelming enough for teacher and resident alike, I have discovered through fifteen years of clinical teaching and supervision, not to mention some reading along the way, that unconscious factors in teacher, resident, and staff alike constantly reframe all that we see and do, setting limits upon our clinical capacities and judgment (Smith 1984, 1986; Smith and Stein 1987). Physicians and social scientists alike are for the most part trained nowadays to pay greater attention to context, defined as the world out there of the patient and family. Our professional education, building upon our earliest family experiences, directs our attention almost exclusively *outward*. "Context" has come to mean exclusively "out there." Yet, if we have learned anything from the near century of contributions from psychoanalysts and others influenced by psychoanalytic insights (cf. Freud 1910:144–45; Balint 1957; Binion 1981; deMause 1982; Devereux 1967; Katz 1984; La Barre 1978; Stein 1985c; Stein and Apprey 1985, 1987), we know that we are part of the very context that we observe and in which we wish clinically or didactically to intervene. By systematically understanding the process, dynamics, meaning of observation, and intervention itself, we become more aware of where we stand and why, and become thereby liberated from inner compulsions to take theoretical and clinical stands one way and only one way. That, of course, is what Balint groups are all about.

"Context" and "doing ethnography" are thus accounts of the interplay of our various stories about ourselves and one another—not just interactional or altogether objective narratives. The need to add the psychodynamic dimension to understanding the physician or teacher behind the assessment and intervention, impressed itself on me—not from doctrine, reading, or formal training—but from day-to-day experiences in clinical teaching and supervision. It was these that sent me back to the books—and to clinical exploration with my self as the subject—in order to understand what and where all context was located.

Countless applied ethnographically oriented or medical anthropology papers, presentations, and workshops on clinical work and teaching have as their subject or focus the world of the patient, of the family, or of the patient's community (e.g., the home, the neighborhood, lay healers, ethnicity, occupational network, and the like; e.g., Kleinman 1980; Harwood 1981). This chapter adopts this ethnographic, contextual frame of reference to the world of biomedicine: e.g., the family-medicine resident and teacher and, to a degree, the medical and physician's associate (P.A.) student and the graduate student in occupational medicine (see also Hahn and Gaines 1985; Stein 1985b). It focuses on the cultural ambience of medicine—one that includes medical and administrative staff, institutional culture, and supralocal influences on medical curriculum and practice. It explores what some of the best teaching contexts for behavioral science might be, and identifies issues of values, status, power, roles, competing priorities, etc., that constantly reframe the official subject matter in these settings.

The remainder of this chapter is presented in three sections: (1) a description of the experiences that led to my elaboration of the ethnographic model; (2) an illustration of the model's application in my current teaching settings; and (3) a discussion of how the ethnographic teaching model can be used to impart the applied anthropologist's "uncomfortable knowledge" (Colson 1985:195). This chapter is the product of fifteen years of development and refinement of an ethnographic approach to clinical teaching, first in the Department of Psychiatry, Meharry Medical College, Nashville, Tennessee (1972–78), and later in the Department of Family Medicine at the University of Oklahoma Health Sciences Center (1978– present). Most recently, my clinical teaching has occurred in several locales: (1) a community-based residency training program at the Enid Family Medicine Clinic, located ninety miles northwest of Oklahoma City, where I have coordinated the behavioral science curriculum since 1978, traveling there some forty-four Fridays per year; (2) a community-based residency training program at the Shawnee Family Medicine Clinic, located thirty-eight miles east of the Oklahoma City tertiary care center, at which program I coordinated behavioral science teaching between 1979 and the program's close in mid-1985, traveling there some twenty-four Mondays per year; (3) an annual graduate course (for M.D.s and P.A.s) in "Behavioral Sciences in Occupational Medicine," which I have offered since 1980; and (4) case conferences, Balint groups (at which psychological difficulties in physician/patient and physician/physician/staff/institution relationships are discussed), faculty advisory meetings with residents, and resident consultations in the Oklahoma City family medicine program (since 1978).

FROM CRISIS TO TECHNIQUE

The psychoanalytically informed ethnographic approach to clinical teaching and supervision (Stein 1982b, 1985b, 1985c; Stein and Apprey 1985, 1987) is the product of what I regard as a *personal* and *professional crisis,* or rather, a *series of crises.* Very simply, *what* I had to offer (content) and *how* I wanted and was prepared to offer it (including how I was trained to do so) were frequently received with little enthusiasm, if not rejected. Many medical, P.A., and public health graduate students, psychiatry and family-medicine residents, and faculty—including behavioral scientists of many disciplines—have been, at most, lukewarm about what I felt most ardently. This seemed ironic, since what I thought I was teaching implemented at least the officially promulgated stand of these colleagues and their disciplines: contextual thinking, teaching, research, clinical practice, with special emphasis on learning about the family, community, and culture of the patient in order to learn to work within the latter contexts as well as the biomedical. Yet often, in practice (as opposed to theory = ideal) we had no overlapping view of my subject matter while at other times, they had preconceived, fixed notions of what my subject matter should be and how I should teach it.

Part of the intercultural communication problem lay in the conceptual disparity between the *biomedical* model, with its body-bound organ systems, and the broader, more inclusive, integrative biopsychosocial model. Beyond the mere *cognitive* difference, I soon learned, was the frequent use of biomedical theory, doctrine, and practice as individually and institutionally sanctioned *defense mechanisms.* This fact gradually prompted me to focus on "countertransference" as an ongoing research-cum-teaching project (as did Balint, Devereux, La Barre, and Katz). There was thus not only *unfamiliarity* between their world and mine, but the medical worldview was itself used as a form of *resistance* to learning the material I had aspired to teach about the subjective world of patients—and patients' families and personal networks—in sickness and in health. The objectivity and the professional distance of the medical model were used to keep at bay and compartmentalize what I was trying to bring closer and to integrate. The subjective world of a patient's suffering, and the prospect of both personalizing that dimension and incorporating it into medical practice, were often experienced more as a *threat* than as an *opportunity*.

There were other disparities as well. While contributions from, say, biochemists, pathologists, internists, and surgeons (the so-called hard and basic medical sciences) tend to be accepted in medical education as high status, specialist viewpoints—with a considerable range of eclecticism allowed; I have found that for the behavioral or social scientist little such tolerance is shown. Simply put, whereas biomedical and medical administrative professionals tend to accept without screening what biomedical specialists have to say, these same colleagues work on the basis of what might be called a folk psychology or sociology that serves as the basis of acceptance for what the behavioral scientist would like to say or do. Mere training, degree, or publication does not automatically confer acceptability of a behavioral scientist's ideas presented to a medical or residency group. Rather, medical colleagues often assume that everybody knows behavioral science in a way that everybody *does not* know surgery or obstetrics. Therefore, I am not perceived to be a scientist in the same sense as those in the basic and clinical sciences, nor am I automatically entitled to have a forum to present or "profess" them.

Lest the reader think that this is flagrant censorship, I would add that, frustrating and demoralizing as this process is, it is more subtle and insidious than censorship. Such biomedical and wider cultural resistance has compelled me to rethink both how I teach and what I teach. Paradoxically, perhaps, my goals and ideals are not compromised. The closest analogue to this approach is, perhaps obviously, that of psychoanalytic psychotherapy in which resistance, transference, and countertransference play a decisive role in the educational process.

I could not in good conscience promote what I was often expected to provide for medical students or residents, e.g., the popular disease-entity model of alcoholism, along with brief techniques to cure anorexia nervosa and obesity. Further, few others thought the complexly textured systems thinking and working that I thought essential to good medical practice practical or even possible—although many residents have gradually adopted the approach while protesting that it required too much time and money. I have learned to monitor my own ambitions, disappointments, guilt, and rage to avoid making medical students and colleagues into extensions of my wishes and fantasies rather than accepting them as real persons. In graduate training, I had been taught to expect to walk into a class—*my* class—and give a lecture or offer a seminar. The crisis confronted me with an overwhelming sense of limitation, inadequacy, rage, and failure—feelings that physicians, too, flee from with terror. From this I learned empathy for a *common* plight: their wish for activism differed from mine in specific content only, not in aim. The psychoanalytically-informed ethnographic approach to clinical teaching emerged as my resolution of the crisis—a method in which insight into myself became a crucial tool for my capacity to work within the medical world (see Stein and Apprey 1985, 1987).

Bronislaw Malinowski learned about the Trobriand Islanders by living among them, by getting to know them on their own terms, by becoming incorporated—at least to a degree—into their world. Similarly, I have learned the world of family medicine, and how, when, and where to teach "behavioral sciences" to family medicine residents, to occupational medicine physicians, and to graduate students by spending a considerable amount of time over the years getting to know them and their interests, priorities, expectations, and training ambience—in a sense, by virtually living among them. I teach largely by attempting to reframe or sculpt my agenda and contents to their context. I try to reach them in their world and with their world, and not just to ask them to heed mine.

I have learned this the hard way, through many disappointments, defeats, and outright revolutions by residents and faculty colleagues when I had unwittingly attempted to do too much—as in lecture content or readings—"my way" (see Stein 1983). My error, one not altogether my own, was my initial assumption that I was to teach *as if* I were in an academic environment, as if new knowledge or ways of clinical thinking and feeling were prized, and therefore that my task was to teach "my subject." I have subsequently learned through experience to teach even a highly academic seminar—e.g., an annual graduate level course called "Behavioral Sciences in Occupational Medicine"—*by making the interests, occupational choices, in short, the lives, of those taking the course as an intrinsic part of the subject matter of the course itself.* I teach immersion in clinical context by first immersing myself in the contexts of the clinicians whom I am teaching.

For instance, a typical Friday consists of a twelve-to-fifteen-hour workday, that begins with a one and one-half hours drive from my home to a clinic site in Enid, Oklahoma. At 7:30 A.M., I participate in "sit down" hospital grand rounds, continue with consultations with staff and physicians, a noon conference lecture, scheduling of community speakers, and a return in late afternoon or early evening bearing the clinic mail and financial paperwork for the department's main office. Much of my time is spent in working with faculty and clinical/administrative staff to help prepare the residency teaching *context* that is hardly limited to me.

The hallmark of the ethnographic approach to clinical (or any) teaching is the fact that I conduct ongoing fieldwork or research in the teaching context(s) itself as an intrinsic part of teaching about the content or subject of the lecture, seminar, or grand rounds. For me *ethnographic* connotes simultaneously the ethnographic content or focus of the *topic* and *the very process of teaching about that topic.* I do not simply ask residents or graduate students to be better aware of the contexts from which their patients come. Rather, I try to be constantly aware of—and inquire into—the multiple contexts the students or residents themselves bring, together with the very context of the group dynamics or "group culture" of the classroom or clinic seminar itself. Teaching *about* fieldwork (clinical supervision of taking a patient's life situation seriously) and teaching *as* fieldwork (clinical supervision as taking the resident's beliefs and responses as seriously as I ask him or her to take those of the patient) are two sides of the same coin. The parallel to psychoanalysis—with its training analysis in which the observed analysand learns to become self-observant and hence to observe better—is precise, although I did not consciously model my ethnographic teaching approach from it.

In short, the ethnographic approach to clinical teaching is an attitude congruent with the tenets of applied anthropology: attempting to effect change, to accomplish specific tasks, etc., within the context of a community or culture's values, power structure, and beliefs, and within the framework of understanding that culture's built-in contradictions and ambivalences. It is only our—and certainly my—illusion and wish that medical students, residents, or graduate students have no agendas other than the one we wish to impart to them that prevents us from utilizing an ethnographic style in our very teaching. Students' and residents' agendas, conscious and unconscious, of course affect how they learn, selectively learn, or fail to learn the very context sensitivity that is our subject matter.

For example, in the graduate seminar "Behavioral Sciences in Occupational Medicine: An Ethnographic Approach," which I have offered annually for six years, I have long had exceptional administration (M.D. and P.A.) support for keeping academic standards high (e.g., there is much reading, fieldwork, and a term paper). These same administrators—two of whom were formerly graduate students in the course—likewise appreciate the fact that I have always tailored the seminar to the clinical and administrative world for which the physician and physician's associate graduate students are preparing themselves. In addition to a "generic" ethnographic tailoring of the course, I inquire early in each seminar into the interests, career plans, and work-related experiences of each graduate student, and help each to select a field site/project on some topic that is already of interest to that student.

One student, for instance, was an avid advocate of smoking cessation programs, having lost a beloved grandfather some years ago to emphysema. He elected to conduct an ethnographic study of smoking behavior, relationships, and meanings among employees in a local family medicine clinic. In addition to wanting them to stop smoking, he was gradually able to take an interest in their world, in which smoking played some part. Another student, angry about the extent to which Veterans Administration hospitals seemed to foster dependency in their patients, conducted an ethnographic study on the interplay between the family, occupational, and medical worlds in the life of one VA patient (see chapter 5 of this volume). My approach to this course illustrates my belief that, by incorporating the students' interests and experiences and goals into the very topic matter, I enhance their willingness to learn patently alien subject matter. (The course is invariably offered at the end of a "hard science"–dominated Masters in Public Health curriculum in occupational health, the core of which consists of courses in engineering-oriented industrial hygiene, clinical medicine, and health administration.)

After offering this seminar for several years, I stumbled upon the fact that the graduate students, seasoned clinicians in the "real" world, had received only book-learning and examining-room experience in their occupational-medicine training. I had assumed that they had, in other courses, been surfeited with field trips to actual work sites. I was wrong, and they in fact yearned for such experience. As a result, in recent years, we regularly have had lengthy tours of a silk-screening advertising plant, an air force base, and a plant that manufactures anhydrous ammonia and urea for fertilizers—implementing, in a phrase, family and occupational medicine's doctrine of community-oriented primary care. For each class, these field trips are deeply transforming experiences.

Thus, the ethnographic approach is simultaneously (1) a strategy to introduce academic material and standards into what is in many respects a functionally nonacademic environment, and (2) an effort to take seriously the world that the graduate students, residents, and medical students bring to their training and the world of clinical or administrative practice for which I am preparing them. I do not simply teach "a subject"; I teach students. The evolution of my relationship with them becomes the evolution of my introduction of specific subject matter.

The ethnographic approach to clinical teaching extends even to the choice of subject matter itself. Often I cannot simply declare that "I want to teach such and such to medical students and residents because it is important for them to learn it, or because anthropologists/psychologists . . . deem it important." Rather, I must often *embed my own curriculum agendas in medically* (which is to say, *culturally*) *acceptable language and forms*—which is no different from applied anthropology in intercultural or international work.

THE ETHNOGRAPHIC TRAINING MODEL IN A FAMILY MEDICINE SETTING

In this section, I enumerate a series of "emic" categories (viz., those constructed within the culture of family medicine) that affect my behavioral science teaching in family medicine. For each category I offer brief vignettes that illustrate how the ethnographic approach is implemented. Although this typology is specific to the Oklahoma family-medicine setting, I strongly suspect that much, if not all, of it could be construed as *etic*-ally transposable to other organizational settings. Two worksheets—figures 6.1 and 6.2—are provided both to summarize the narrative and to serve as a matrix with which the reader can assess ethnographically his or her clinical work setting.

Identifying Contextual Opportunities and Limitations in Clinical Teaching

Whom to teach? My official job description lists me as behavioral science consultant to teach clinical behavioral science to family medicine residents. However, my informally negotiated role over the years has expanded to consulting/counseling with medical/administrative faculty and staff, and assisting in clinicwide mo-

Whom to teach?

What to teach?

Where to teach (spatial considerations)?

When to teach (timing)?

How to teach?

Who should do the teaching?

Value considerations (What is most prized, disdained, tabooed?) in the institution?

Authority and *power* considerations?

How to get residents to *read* behavioral science articles, chapters, books?

Identification of key *issues* that should be addressed and
taught? Who defines educational *agendas*? What are the
metaissues (within and beyond the group) that frame or
qualify teaching issues? What may and may not be said?
What are the implicit and explicit group rules that affect
teaching/learning activities in family medicine?

Competing teacher *roles* (e.g., practitioner, administrator,
teacher, researcher, scholar) and effect on teaching?

Integration of community in the teaching process?

Culturally acceptable or standard *teaching techniques* or
methods?

Teacher's own *values* and *expectations* and *limitations*? What will
I *not* do?

Training evaluation and *outcome* studies? *Sequence* and *hierarchy*
of learning?

Figure 6.1   *Identifying contextual opportunities and limitations in clinical
teaching*

What are my goals, objectives, agendas, values, expectations, beliefs, attitudes, out-of-awareness issues? With *whom* do I think I teach best (including "no one")? In which *settings* do I think I teach best?

What are the goals, objectives, agendas, values, expectations, beliefs, attitudes, out-of-awareness issues of my work colleagues, superiors, staff, residents, medical students, P.A. students (graduate and undergraduate)? With whom do they think I teach best (including "no one")? In which *settings* do they think I teach best?

How can a setting (physical, people) *facilitate* me in teaching? What are the pertinent roles, rules, values, leaders (formal vs. informal sources of influence), settings, etc.? Who should I try to work with? Where should I best work to accomplish my/their/our aims?

How does a setting (physical, people) *interfere* with my ability to teach? Can (If so, how) these differences in roles, rules, values, expectations, priorities, be negotiated, conflict made explicit, compromises or trade-offs reached, etc.? What cannot be talked about?

Figure 6.2   Ethnographically oriented clinical-teaching worksheet

rale-building and community-organization work. When the closing of one clinic was imminent, I spent much time visiting with
and counseling individuals and the clinic group over issues of
mourning, rage, helplessness, etc., which contributed to resident
education indirectly, but which addressed programwide unrest.

What to teach? There is a constant interplay between what I wish to
teach, program needs, and the timing of what the residents are
most receptive to learn (see Stein and Grant 1986). There are
also supralocal, nationally mandated topic areas in family medicine that I attempt to integrate into the behavioral science curriculum: e.g., family dynamics, community-oriented primary care,
occupational medicine, and geriatrics. My greatest challenge is to
interpolate these within a sense of the whole, and not to contribute further to fragmentation.

   Although we are mandated to prepare physicians for per-
sonalistic and rural practices—urban, tertiary-care, high-tech,
procedure-centered, and hospital-based practice tends to pre-
dominate. Although I make regular presentations on rural medical issues, I recognize that this topic is of largely ceremonial
value. I persist because part of our patient population is geo-
graphically rural (to be distinguished somewhat from those urban dwellers who retain rural values and worldviews). At the
same time, I balance my own ambitions by accepting and working within residents' and faculties' values and priorities: e.g., by
raising contextual questions in case conferences and other regular department teaching functions. I also have adopted a very
long-term view of teaching "success."

Where to teach (spatial considerations)? Given residents' busy schedules and priorities, it is often more practical to ask them to see
whole families when taking care of a hospitalized patient (e.g.,
family conference on the ward, outside the surgical suite) rather
than to insist that they bring the whole family into the outpatient
clinic.

   I do much official teaching in the clinic conference room
(behavioral science noon conference), and much individual consulting of residents and staff in my office (adjacent to the conference room). Likewise, much informal teaching takes place
through "hallway" consultations, discussions in resident's offices,
and around the nurses' station, i.e., in the residents' own terri-
tory.

When to teach (timing)? During the past ten years, when I have been teaching family medicine residents, I have abstained from taking vacation in the months of July and August. These are residents' initial months in internship or community-based residency programs, times when they are most receptive to orientation to the clinic and community organization: that is, times when they are most eager to learn about a subject I wish to teach.

Some years ago, residents asked me at Christmastime to schedule a lecture about getting smokers, alcoholics, and obese people to learn to control themselves. When I presented the topic in January, few attended; the residents asked me to reschedule for the next month. On that occasion, when I gave the formal lecture, they collectively *thanked* me for not having talked about that topic during the Thanksgiving–Christmas–Superbowl Sunday period (even though they had asked me to do so, railing at their inability to control their patients), since they wanted to feel free to eat and drink during the cultural saturnalia. I used this timing to talk about culture-wide ambivalence between self-control and self-indulgence, their ambivalent role as societal policeman, their wish to be out of control yet to control others, and the timing of these issues in the annual cycle. The ostensible issues of difficult scheduling and difficult patients were revealed to be physician issues as well.

I noted earlier that I attend early morning "sit down" grand rounds in the Enid program. At these conferences residents and M.D. faculty discuss diagnostic and management issues related to hospitalized patients. Although I say little during grand rounds, I learn the crucial clinical, programmatic, and community concerns from the past week. I gain access to the cases, diseases, and management problems that occupy faculty, residents, and staff. Immediately following rounds, I often seek out one or two residents, make a comment on some psychosocial aspect of one of *their* cases, and offer to talk with them later in the day about it. These conversations often turn into a consultation, sometimes into a visit with the resident to the patient's bedside for an interview, or occasionally into a supervised session with the patient in the clinic. Likewise, these impromptu discussions often become the basis for a behavioral-science conference topic on a future Friday.

Instead of insisting on teaching solely with *my* cases, I take an interest in the residents and *their* cases, endeavoring to make some of my theoretical or clinical points with *their* material— material in which they already have a vested interest. "What" is teachable often depends upon "when" and "where" it is taught. Ostensibly, "my" time is the Friday noon behavioral-science conference; "their" time is grand rounds. Yet, I get crucial ideas and cases from the residents and medical faculty, and weave them into the behavioral science conferences. Indeed, once a month a conference is devoted entirely to some diagnostic topic or case in which a resident is interested, or some topic the resident wishes to review for a future in-service or boards examination.

Residents often discuss personal, family, and role problems as well as case-related problems with me in conversations that spontaneously and fortuitously reveal meanings of and solutions to more strictly clinical problems that we dealt with previously. It is from such consultations and counseling that I was led to the centrality of countertransference in medical education and practice (Stein 1985c; Stein and Apprey 1985).

Most American primary, secondary, and postsecondary education is cumulative rather than episodic. Students enrolled in a course are expected to attend for the duration; the instructor can sequentially develop or build a topic over time, basing later material upon earlier. In teaching family-medicine residents I cannot take these structural assumptions for granted; residents routinely must be available for their numerous and fluctuating clinical obligations. Because many of the residents are rarely regular participants in the behavioral sciences conference over the weeks, it is difficult to build on earlier topics; the lecturer or presenter cannot assume that the residents have all been exposed to the same material. Put simply, I rarely can pick up where I left off the last time, since many members of the resident group will now be different. Moreover, because second- and third-year family medicine residents attend mostly conferences in programs with which I am affiliated, much repetition is inevitable.

Many interns, residents, and medical faculty abide by the unspoken rule that "No medical conference for which a meal is not provided is worth attending." The intellectual content or fare of a medical lecture or seminar is for many secondary to whether one was first lavishly fed. Many feel indignant and deprived if a speaker does not first nourish his or her audience before speaking. Faculty and residents alike make considerable effort to have conferences sponsored by pharmaceutical companies. In the face of such culinary claims, the beleaguered behavioral scientist who can only offer "food for thought," and who asks interns and residents to bring their own lunches, is at a distinct disadvantage. Over the years, many residents have inquired of me shortly prior to my conferences, not "What's the topic today?" but "Is lunch provided?"

How to teach? I have learned to work within this value hierarchy and competing commitments, by (1) using residents' cases and interests as the foundation for building my lectures, (2) scheduling residents once a month to present their own behavioral science case or topic, (3) consulting (often in the hallway, near the nurses' station) with residents individually about difficult cases, (4) conducting ad hoc, brief personal counseling or supportive therapy, and (5) seeing patients or families with residents in the clinic or hospital. In short, many of my most successful "behavioral science" roles vis-à-vis residents closely approximate roles the residents have negotiated with faculty physicians.

Although I often prefer to present a didactic-style lecture, one that covers unfamiliar aspects of illness, residents and other faculty tend to prefer case-, fact-, and procedure-oriented conferences that both tell them concretely what to do and engage them actively (versus being passive listeners). "Style" itself is a cultural value. My approach has become heavily case-oriented (particularly drawing upon residents' own grand-rounds case presentations and interests), whereby the meaning of *doing* is subtly examined.

Who should do the teaching? "What do *I* want to teach?" often differs markedly from "To whom do the residents listen?" or "Whom do they respect?" I work closely with program faculty/ staff to find out what some of the natural associations are and to promote collaboration with a given resident on a behavioral science subject where the residents are already receptive to specific faculty/staff member(s). Not only do I not try to "do it all" myself, I try to foster a program atmosphere in which the environment becomes the teacher.

Value considerations (What is most prized, disdained, tabooed?) in the institution? The polarities of doing/thinking, action/ reflection, aggression/passivity organize medical education and practice. The image of physician or teacher is that of doer, intervenor, curer, warrior, and military winner. Residents are most amenable to feeling and reflection when some form of "doing" fails. This nether side of medicine is dealt with in case-oriented conferences about "difficult" patients and vexing resident/institution relations. I try to work within the residents' biomedical value hierarchy and to help them understand the meaning and consequences of their value choices.

Authority and *power* considerations? Within family medicine, I try to avoid competing with the medical and behavioral-science hierarchy. Most of my influence is informal and unofficial and is thus nonthreatening to others' vested interests and position. Over time, paradoxically, such a position has accrued considerable authority.

How to get residents to *read* behavioral-science articles, chapters, books? I have had little success in assigning readings for my behavioral-science conferences; better success has been achieved by suggesting readings (sparingly and only occasionally) for the residents' Journal Club, or by recommending reading (or giving handouts) on topics related to a problem a resident associates with a specific patient.

Identification of *key issues* that should be addressed and taught? Who defines educational agendas? What are the *metaissues* (within and beyond the group) that frame or qualify teaching issues? What may and may not be said? What are the implicit and explicit group rules that affect teaching/learning activities in family medicine?

Key issues are closely tied to goals. The question is "Whose"?—residents', mine, other behavioral science or medical faculty's, the urban-based department's, the community-based residency program's, those of national family medicine organizations? These are often divergent. What *may* be taught, what topics are given curriculum time, are highly political issues that are in turn shaped by group process and by the personal meaning of specific theories and treatment modalities. Some years ago, the department's overarching emphasis was on "family systems"; drug abuse, occupational medicine, geriatrics, and clinical decision making have recently been added. For several years, the hegemony of certain theories (e.g., Minuchin family-structural model, alcoholism disease model) and highly directive, symptom-focused treatment models have often made it difficult for me to find forums in which to teach my own views of clinical relationships and alcoholism (see Stein 1982a, 1985a).

Competing teacher *roles* (e.g., practitioner, administrator, teacher, researcher, scholar) and effect on teaching? Being informally integrated into the Enid and Shawnee, Oklahoma, medical communities, I have always felt welcome to visit and interview hospitalized patients together with residents. When the main department office asked that I seek formal hospital privileges at the tertiary care campus, it asked me to do likewise in these community settings. I was quietly told in the community programs that I already have them so long as I don't request them formally—in which latter case the request would have to be declined to avoid setting a precedent. I notified the departmental office of these unspoken rules, and it agreed to accept the informal agreement as sufficient.

Although teaching is ostensibly of the highest institutional value, it is the least rewarded and is accorded relatively low value and support for preparing instructional materials. Income production, grantsmanship, "hard" science research are most prized and rewarded. The charge of not doing enough is frequently made, even when there are "not enough hours in the day" to do more that would in any event compromise one's teaching obligations and commitments.

With respect to behavioral-scientist status and role issues in family-medicine settings, consider the question "What's in a name?" What is my identity from my viewpoint, and as ascribed by others? What do I wish to label myself, and what do other medical colleagues label me? What overlap is possible—with what dignity, and at what price? I am on the faculty, yet interns and residents often use the term *faculty* to denote physicians only. By profession, I am a medical anthropologist, psychoanalytic anthropologist, and psychohistorian. Over the years, many medical and administrative colleagues and patients—especially in community training settings—have labeled me variously as "psychiatrist," "psychologist," "behavioral scientist," "family therapist," "like a social worker," "our shrink," and so forth. Although flattered, I have for ethical and legal reasons politely but firmly declined the psychiatrist, psychologist, and social worker encomia. Such protestation is usually to little avail, for these labels remain the only frames of reference in which my very presence and function make sense. I rarely correct them anymore.

Anthropology, with whatever qualifier, for most connotes archaeology, the remote past, and peoples far more primitive than they wish to view themselves. Too much emphasis on psycho-anything in this geographic region conjures images of sin, Satan, and the projective accusation that one might be guilty, crazy, or out of control. During my decade thus far in Oklahoma, *behavioral scientist* seems to be the term that has the best fit between my own and others' fantasies—role expectations of me; it is also the most descriptive and neutral. Nonetheless, role boundaries and status anxiety remain a perpetual problem; I must constantly renegotiate and try to clarify status and role. The "liminal" or in-between role and status of family medicine is a painfully familiar chronic uncertainty among family physicians—especially in academic centers. Yet, in that gray zone of role and status ambiguity, there is much room for creativity. It is the flip side of the time and energy it requires to define and account for oneself almost constantly.

Integration of community in the teaching process? Outpatient, community-based care is a family medicine ideal, one that makes home visits "natural." Yet family medicine's emulation of high-tech, hospital-based, problem-focused subspecialties makes it difficult for residents to take the former ideal very seriously. Efforts are made to interest residents in the community as a means toward practice building (see Snider and Stein 1987). In practice management training, residents are encouraged to develop key community informants, and to make themselves visible through service to schools, business organizations, and community service agencies.

Culturally acceptable or standard teaching *techniques* or *methods*? For several years when "family systems" was the prevailing ideology, the "genogram" (similar to anthropologists' kinship diagrams) was a widely used instrument for teaching about families. I adapted it as a somewhat safe, distant way to help residents to examine their own and patients' emotionally volatile or taboo subjects.

Teacher's own *values* and *expectations* and *limitations*? What will I *not* do? There are limits to my cultural accommodation, that is, to what I will do (see also Devereux 1967). In adapting the ethnographic approach to clinical teaching, I refuse to serve as "provider" of approaches that oversimplify issues or demean any or all participants. I try to help interns, residents, and faculty colleagues tolerate anxiety over complexity and ambiguity.

Training evaluation and *outcome* studies? *Sequence* and *hierarchy* of learning? All educational programs have evaluations to study the outcome of the training process. Family medicine is no exception. We conduct ongoing short-term evaluations of resident performance in behavioral science and other areas. These culturally standardized approaches cannot be circumvented, since they are widely regarded as "hard" science and therefore reliable. However, I urge colleagues that these be supplemented by more impressionistic data generated by residents and graduate physicians on their own timetables. Time and experience seem important criteria by which residents and ex-residents evaluate behavioral science.

Although behavioral sciences are a regular part of family medicine residents' three year training, residents characteristically seek first to get their biomedical facts "down cold," to hone their differential diagnostic and procedure skills, and to be accepted in the eyes of their physician colleagues and preceptors. Often it is only after they have completed their residency and have been in practice a year or two *and* feel comfortable, competent, and secure in their biomedical knowledge and skills that they can permit themselves to recognize the utility of their behavioral science training. Thus their long-term evaluation is often discrepant with their culturally accepted short-term one.

CONCLUSION: "UNCOMFORTABLE KNOWLEDGE"
AND THE ETHNOGRAPHIC TEACHING MODEL

In her 1985 Malinowski Award address, Elizabeth Colson summarized the collective experience of many applied anthropologists since early in the twentieth century. The applied social sciences operate "in a charged political arena where the accuracy of information [is] assessed by the degree to which it supported established positions" (1985:182)—positions, I might add, not only in medicine but the social/behavioral sciences as well. Colson continues: "It is a common charge that the social sciences, including anthropology, are unable to produce results in the form of generalizable principles that can be applied to particular cases. In fact, this has not been our primary problem. . . . Our problem arises rather from the fact that our research challenges what others want to believe; our problem lies in obtaining an audience that will listen when the information is not palatable" (1985:193). She concludes by saying that "what we have is uncomfortable knowledge, the kind of knowledge that challenges established cliches and puts in question accepted solutions, and so those who champion them" (1985:195).

This "uncomfortable knowledge" is often precisely, at least in content if not in its implications, *the very kind of knowledge requested by the organization in the first place.* Officially, perhaps also in the group or institutional ideal, medicine wants the information that has been produced and offered by such academic disciplines as anthropology. Unofficially, perhaps in the competing, often implicit, group or institutional ideals and agendas, medicine largely discounts or repudiates the very information it has solicited. For instance, within the profession and discipline of family medicine, teaching and research about the doctor-patient relationship occupies a high priority in the official self-image of this primary care specialty. Many regard psychoanalyst Michael Balint, originator of the "Balint groups" on doctor-patient relationships in England, as one of family medicine's ancestral luminaries. Nonetheless, some years ago one faculty member, citing what he called our "corporate mission" in family-centered research and medical care, questioned the propriety of my study of the topic of countertransference. What had it to do with building the family systems ideological infrastructure of our discipline and institution?—he challenged. When science becomes the handmaiden of careerism, commercialism, power, and doctrine, it forsakes the right to be deemed science.

I have only slowly and reluctantly learned that a discipline's or an institution's *avowed* interest in a topic does not necessarily coincide with its *actual* interest or priority. To comply with the ostensible message or injunction is often to violate the tacit one that cannot be avowed. Family medicine is not exempt from the swift national currents of commercialism, social Darwinism, "technologism," survivalism, and minimalism (see Carlyon 1984; Becker 1987; Stephens 1984a, 1984b; Stein and Hill 1984). Nationalism and nuclearism, too, help set an ominous tone that makes the pursuit of clinical intimacy, depth, and breadth seem little worth the risk.

Discussions of "bridging the gap" between behavioral sciences and biomedicine infrequently introduce the concept of social control to explain why integration remains—after some five decades of effort—so elusive. Ideally, we would like to believe that conflicts between various clinical worldviews (e.g., several family systems theories and models of therapy, biomedical specialty models, individual psychotherapy models, etc.) are resolved by scientific discussion and debate, and a large portion of goodwill. In reality such conflict is often solved by leaders and groups who use positions of authority and official power to differentially advance or enforce certain clinical worldviews. For instance, advocates of a favored medical theory might be given more hours of seminar/classroom time to teach than adherents of less favored theories; likewise, advocates of a favored medical theory might be given greater secretarial and more advanced technological support to disseminate those types of ideas faster than the work of researchers or clinicians who espouse less favored theories.

In our widely touted postindustrial, information/service society, the issue of social control regarding information access, production, and status is rarely addressed. Clearly, however—with apologies to George Orwell—some information is more equal than others. This has been my personal experience as a psychoanalytically oriented behavioral scientist in family medicine, and the experience of family physicians in the larger "family" of medical specialties. I think for instance, of family physician Dr. G. Gayle Stephens's erstwhile journal, *Continuing Education for the Family Physician (CEFP)*, one that I regard as having been editorially courageous, but one that many medical and behavioral science colleagues and residents have regarded as a second-class, throw-away magazine, not clinical enough and certainly not high status enough. Despite Dr. Stephens's efforts, *CEFP* was not listed in *Index Medicus*.

Several years ago, a senior medical colleague wrote me a highly congratulatory letter about an article on the doctor-patient relationship that had recently appeared in *CEFP*. He said that he was writing a paper on a similar subject, and wanted to cite my ideas; however, he continued, the editor(s) of the kind of journal(s) for which he was writing would look askance at his citing an article published in *CEFP*. Was there any chance that I had published similar ideas in a more legitimate, mainstream, medical journal? he inquired. My reply was—I prefer to believe—more indignant and resoundingly self-righteous than I would probably now write. However, the issue was clearly less *what* the ideas were than the status of *where* they were published. Ideas are acceptable only insofar as they are born and reared on the correct ideological and status side of the railroad tracks.

"Uncomfortable knowledge" conveys to the observer valuable information about a group that it already knows, at some level, about itself but cannot tolerate to integrate into its group identity. That is, it cannot tolerate consciously and affectively to know this information about itself. Paradoxically, heresy's unwelcome truths are perceived to be more dangerous than the official fiction—family myth or group fantasy—that must be sustained at all costs. As an applied anthropologist, I not only have the task of finding ways to deal with the political and economic vested interests of those with whom I work but I must be able to acknowledge and to some degree to work within the inevitable limitations set by (1) people's *ambivalence* about their own culture and about their own avowed values; (2) people's tendency to *split* between a good image of their own group identity and a bad image of alternate, outside identities, referred to by Erikson as the "negative identity" (1968); and (3) people's *narcissistic* investment of values, roles, ideals, and the like, that is, their incorporation into the core of the self and its regulation. These unwelcome realities remind me of limitations to my own idealism and ambition for inducing or fostering change. They reevoke my own ambivalences, splits, and countershaming self-protective maneuvers, ones that mirror and intensify those of the group that does not welcome my findings or interests.

In recent writings on the psychology of international relations, a number of authors (Davidson and Montville 1980–81; Montville in press; Saunders 1984; Stein 1987b; Volkan 1986) have proposed a distinction between Track I and Track II diplomacy. Track I is the official, public, ideological, often rancorous and polarizing dance of policy-making and position-taking, Track II is the unofficial, informal, more private, relatively spontaneous, and quiet initiatives by lower-echelon officials and private citizens who search for rapprochement, reconciliation, common ground, or areas of overlapping interests. When working at their best, Track I leaders, amidst their bravura, tacitly delegate to Track II explorers what they themselves cannot do or say; Track II workers provide Track I leaders with alternative visions of the world and of the possible, serving as unofficial sources of new information, as mediators of the familiar and the unfamiliar, of the safe and the dangerous, and as agents of gradual, slow change that does not threaten or undermine the position of Track I leaders.

The ethnographic clinical-teaching method that I have outlined and advocated in this chapter is an example of this Track II principle and strategy as applied to medical education and clinical practice. Its bearers must of necessity occupy a liminal status and role—even when they are assigned formal positions—in the organizational culture. And, as is commonly the case in international affairs as well, when unofficial efforts do become incorporated into official policy and structure, Track I leaders and administrators will usually announce these to be their own initiatives. From the viewpoint of public recognition, Track II–type teaching, clinical practice, and diplomacy is largely thankless: stated differently, much of the sense of self-worth and affirmation of one's role must derive from the intrinsic value of the work and from the gratification that comes from one's more informal contacts. Track II workers in education, as in diplomacy—not unlike psychotherapists—must find ways to feel satisfaction from the facilitating, preparatory, indirect, and usually behind-the-scenes role they occupy—in short, from a long-term view of the process in which they are participating.

The ethnographic training model was born of the repeated crisis of my frustrated belief—and my wish to believe—that official, explicit rules were the principal ones, and that the way to be a good clinical teacher was simply to comply with them. With the ethnographic model, I have learned valuable information about the culture of medicine generally, and of family medicine in particular, that constitutes the "medium" in which clinical behavioral-science teaching takes place. The ethnographic approach helps me to determine (*a*) what is possible (that is, teaching/supervision opportunities), (*b*) limitations on my influence or intervention, and (*c*) how to go about doing the possible. In a sense, this approach transposes and amplifies Kleinman's (1980) "explanatory models" paradigms for physician-patient negotiation to the paradigm between me as clinical teacher and the medical training ambience.

The clinical ethnographic method is only painstakingly acquired and cultivated. It demands long-term commitment to relationships through which knowledge of how to intervene is gained. Further, ethnography for ethnography's sake can lead to endless description and never get around to the *ethnological* task, that is, to the task of building better *theory* about human nature, family and culture, sickness and healing. Clinical ethnography is not arcane, the private property of the discipline of medical anthropology (see Kuzel 1986). It has become for me less a specifically anthropological practice than a way of being in the world, as the existentialists say. At the very least, the ethnographic approach to clinical teaching helps to remind those who use it of the common humanity of all participants in medical education. And if such is the method's only achievement, it is not a small one.

REFERENCES

Balint, M. 1957. *The doctor, his patient, and the illness.* New York: International Universities Press.

Becker, M. H. 1987. The cholesterol saga: Whither health promotion? *Annals of Internal Medicine* 106(4):623–26.

Binion, R. 1981. *Soundings: Psychohistorical and psycholiterary.* New York: Psychohistory Press.

Carlyon, W. H. 1984. Reflections: Disease prevention/health promotion— Bridging the gap to wellness. *Health Values: Achieving High Level Wellness* 8(3):27–30.

Colson, E. 1985. Using anthropology in a world on the move. *Human Organization* 44(3):191–96.

Davidson, W., and J. Montville. 1980–81. Foreign policy according to Freud. *Foreign Policy* 45:145–57.

DeMause, L. 1982. *Foundations of psychohistory.* New York: Creative Roots.

Devereux, G. 1967. *From anxiety to method in the behavioral sciences.* The Hague: Mouton.

De Vos, G. 1966. Toward a cross-cultural psychology of caste behavior. In *Japan's invisible race,* edited by G. De Vos and H. Wagatsuma, 377 ff. Berkeley and Los Angeles: University of California Press.

Erikson, E. H. 1968. *Identity: Youth and crisis.* New York: Norton.

Freud, S. 1910. The future prospects of psycho-analytic therapy. In *The standard edition of the complete psychological works of Sigmund Freud (SE)* 11, translated by J. Strachey, 139–51. London: Hogarth Press, 1957.

GAP Committee on International Relations and H. F. Stein. 1987. *Us and them: The psychology of ethnonationalism.* Group for the Advancement of Psychiatry (GAP) report no. 123. New York: Brunner/Mazel.

Hahn, R. A., and A. D. Gaines, eds. 1985. *Physicians of Western medicine: Anthropological approaches to theory and practice.* Boston: D. Reidel.

Harwood, W., ed. 1981. *Ethnicity and medical care.* Cambridge, Mass.: Harvard University Press.

Katz, J. 1984. *The silent world of doctor and patient.* New York: The Free Press/ Macmillan.

Kleinman, A. 1980. *Patients and healers in the context of culture: An exploration of the borderland between anthropology, medicine, and psychiatry.* Berkeley and Los Angeles: University of California Press.

Kuzel, A. J. 1986. Naturalistic inquiry: An appropriate model for family medicine. *Family Medicine* 18(6):369–74.

La Barre, W. 1978. The clinic and the field. In *The making of psychological anthropology,* edited by G. D. Spindler, 258–99. Berkeley and Los Angeles: University of California Press.

Montville, J. In press. Psychoanalytic enlightenment and the greening of diplomacy. *Journal of the American Psychoanalytic Association.*

Saunders, H. H. 1984. When citizens talk: A look at nonofficial dialogue in relations between nations. *Kettering Review,* Summer:49–55.

Smith, R. C. 1984. Teaching interviewing skills to medical students: The issue of "countertransference." *Journal of Medical Education* 59:582–88.

———. 1986. Unrecognized responses and feelings of residents and fellows during interviews of patients. *Journal of Medical Education* 61:982–84.

Smith, R. C., and H. F. Stein. 1987. A topographical model of clinical decision making and interviewing. *Family Medicine* 19(5):361–63.

Snider, G., and H. F. Stein. 1987. An approach to community assessment in medical practice. *Family Medicine* 19(3):213–19.

Stein H. F. 1982a. Ethanol and its discontents: Paradoxes of inebriation and sobriety in American culture. *Journal of Psychoanalytic Anthropology* 5(4): 355–77.

———. 1982b. The ethnographic mode of teaching clinical behavioral science. In *Clinically applied anthropology: Anthropologists in health science settings*, edited by N. Chrisman and T. Maretzki, 61–82. Boston: D. Reidel.

———. 1983. Lessons of the revolution: A critical event and the contexts of family systems medicine. *Family Systems Medicine* 1(3):31–36.

———. 1985a. Alcoholism as metaphor in American culture: Ritual desecration as social integration. *Ethos* 13(3):195–235.

———. 1985b. Principles of style: A medical anthropologist as clinical teacher. *Medical Anthropology Quarterly* 16(3):64–67.

———. 1985c. *The psychodynamics of medical practice: Unconscious factors in patient care*. Berkeley and Los Angeles: University of California Press.

———. 1985d. Psychological complementarity in Soviet-American relations. *Political Psychology* 6(2):249–61.

———. 1987a. *Developmental time, cultural space: Studies in psychogeography*. Norman: University of Oklahoma Press.

———. 1987b. Encompassing systems: Implications for citizen diplomacy. *Journal of Humanistic Psychology* 27(3):364–84.

Stein, H. F., and M. Apprey. 1985. *Context and dynamics in clinical knowledge*, vol. 1 of the Series in Ethnicity, Medicine, and Psychoanalysis. Charlottesville: University Press of Virginia.

———. 1987. *From metaphor to meaning: Papers in psychoanalytic anthropology*, vol. 2 of the Series in Ethnicity, Medicine, and Psychoanalysis. Charlottesville: University Press of Virginia.

Stein, H. F., and W. D. Grant. 1986. *Behavioral science in family medicine: A program for second and third year family medicine residents*. Kansas City, Mo.: The Society of Teachers of Family Medicine.

Stein, H. F., and R. F. Hill. 1984. American medicine and the enchanted machine. *Continuing Education for the Family Physician* 19(8):428–30.

Stephens, G. G. 1984a. The medical supermarket: Futuristic or decadent? *Continuing Education for the Family Physician* 19(5):243, 245.

———. 1984b. The medical supermarket: Futuristic or decadent? Part 2. *Continuing Education for the Family Physician* 19(11):600–610.

Volkan, V. D. 1986. The narcissism of minor differences in the psychological gap between opposing nations. *Psychoanalytic Inquiry* 6(2):175–91.

Watzlawick, P., J. Beavin, and D. Jackson. 1967. *Pragmatics of Human Communication*. New York: Norton.

CHAPTER 7

Family Diseases and
Family History

HOWARD F. STEIN

By profession, I am a scholar of families and a teacher about families—their members' personalities, their cultural styles, their afflictions, and their histories. As a medical anthropologist, I teach what is often called "behavioral sciences" to resident physicians training in family medicine at a large university in the American Great Plains and supervise these young doctors in many of their encounters with patients and families. Unlocking the significance of family illness is neither easy to do oneself nor is it easy to teach others to do it for themselves. I sometimes despair that the very notion of "taking" an instant medical history, family history, and social history is a noble, if dangerous, illusion.

Families are mostly loathe to yield up to their physicians—let alone to one another—the secrets of their symptoms and diseases. The price of safety from despair is a pall of silence and sorrow that only rarely lifts—and then only for a brief reprieve. Almost all that is displayed within the family and to the world is physical suffering. Genograms, paper-and-pencil self-reports, structural family assessments, and the like—tools of the trade for many family-oriented physicians and therapists—are, at best, points of departure, preliminary scaffolding for what only the edifice of time and relationship can build together. For if the character of personal and family history is crystallized in symptom patterns and sickness behavior, its significance in the unfolding of people's medical history is usually opaque and only gradually—and rarely completely—reveals itself to the patient physician. In *The Psychological Autopsy*, A. D. Weisman and R. K. Kastenbaum (1968) make the important distinction between the biomedical disease people *die with* and the psychological ailment they in fact *die from*. (A poignant use of this interpretive framework in understanding the life, creativity, final illness, and death of composer/conductor Gustav Mahler has been made by Feder [1978].) Such a distinction could profitably be extended to include families as well. Given the present skills and priorities of American biomedicine, it is far easier for physicians to diagnose what people die with than it is for them to identify what people die from.

One family, emigrants in the early 1900s from what used to be called Russian Poland, was rife with hypertension, heart disease, stroke, diabetes, paranoia, and that scourge of curative biomedicine—hypochondriasis. The family had owned and operated a successful tavern and boasted not only fine Talmudic scholars but an ancestral eighteenth-century diplomat who had had access to the ear of the Russian tsar, before whom he had pleaded for the protection and emancipation of Russian Jews. If any Jewish family of those times could consider itself settled and respected—within its own religious community, in the eyes of the surrounding Poles and Russians, and even in the eyes of the authorities—this one could.

In 1881, all of this abruptly changed. With the assassination of the liberal, reformist Tsar Alexander II, and the accession to the Romanov throne of the reactionary Alexander III, governmental decrees and officially sponsored pogroms (massacres) against Jews abrogated the family's hard-won status and security and deprived them of all their property and fortune. Their cultural world now lay in ruins. Murder and pillage, forced relocation and expulsion, became an expectation of their everyday world. Nothing any longer was theirs.

As for many millions of emigrants from eastern and central Europe between 1880 and 1914, the United States became their sanctuary and their new dream—political, economic, religious, familial, all in one. Four of the eighteen children died while still in Europe. One by one, and alternatively several at a time, the long stream of surviving fourteen brothers and sisters, in their teens or younger, came to this country and brought their parents. They began as ragpickers and pushcart peddlers, settling in various towns and cities along a river valley in the eastern United States. In a matter of years, they became enviably prosperous dry goods merchants, tavern owners, and restaurant proprietors. They started a new life in the New World.

But the old life and the Old World did not readily give up the ghost: they haunted the living in life and in death. Feeling oppressed by an autocratic father and the still-fresh memory of persecution, many sought in money and property a security that neither could confer. Their homes often even looked like massive fortresses. They hoarded people, possessions, and profits alike. They rarely could permit themselves or allow their children to enjoy the fruits of their arduous labor. Money was constantly reinvested in real estate, stocks, bonds, and banks—as if they could acquire from America and exact from her what they had been so humiliatingly and devastatingly deprived of in Europe. Accumulations were a bulwark against the tyranny of memory—of losses that could not be acknowledged because they were so painful.

One sister had multiple locks installed on the door to her home. With them she would seal herself off from the outside world. Inside her cavern, bereft of furniture, only a ten-watt light bulb shone. Her home was less a place to live than to hide. She kept almost all of her possessions in the suitcases, trunks, and crates out of which she lived—ready at a moment's notice to shut herself in for a siege or to flee. Only terror was permanent.

Other family members haughtily flaunted their American status by adorning themselves with expensive suits, dresses, shoes, and other attire and by putting themselves and their success on display in synagogue, store, and street alike. The external affluence they showed they hardly felt. Coarse and arrogant in their public demeanor and in their family sanctuary—the two most common modes of relating to others were silence and shouting—they gave no hint of the deep hurt behind their boastful contempt. At least in clothing, financial investments, and real estate, they could dissimulate the demeanor of aristocrats rather than live at the mercy of fickle tsars and peasants.

Beneath their pretenses and genuine successes, life remained a disappointment to them. Perhaps they never knew it consciously—they certainly never articulated it; but they mentally lived as though they were in the wrong place and should have been in another time. Their environment could not measure up to their expectations of it. Unwittingly, they transposed the Old World onto the New World, even as many of them vehemently rejected the Old. No one, nothing, was good enough. Unfulfilled and unfulfillable ambition breeded disgust with themselves, which they turned into contempt for all others. The old life could not—despite all the hard work and conspicuous displays—be coerced back into being. Nor could the family let go of the necessity that it be restored. That necessity, together with the conviction that it was their obligation and right, was transmitted to each new generation. The family sustained and perpetuated itself by the sacred grudge against history that it harbored. It was the duty of the next generation to remain faithful to the grudge and redeem it by reversing history. To dislodge emotionally from the family was to commit the most heinous crime: to give up the hope that the past could be restored. That was the ultimate betrayal of the family trust.

Theirs was a hopeless odyssey: to become nobility in a land where nobility was mostly ridiculed (admiration for the pageantry of British royalty, the ubiquity of football homecoming "kings" and "queens," and bureaucratic hierarchy are all, of course, notable exceptions that betray much *American* secret continuity with the Old World). Their sense of entitlement toward the environment was misplaced. For their conviction that history owed them something was not matched by anything in the rough-and-ready American environment. In one sense, that very different American ambience allowed them to make their considerable American successes. But in another sense, the more important familial one, success in the American sense could never produce the yearned-for success in the old European sense.

Deep in their hearts, they felt themselves to be failures. No matter how well they did here, they felt that they deserved better. It was not that what they *did* did not earn them comfort and security; rather, who they *were* was not, and could not be, recognized. And claims upon history that were not recognized could not be honored, let alone redressed. For all their worldly success, they felt an oppressive sense of shame, for they could not be who they felt they were, and they could not allow themselves to betray the family hope by changing.

One tyrant whose domination they could not overthrow was their father's. Yet, no sooner were his sons and daughters free, American style, than they reinstated the family feudal system when they married and had children. The family was not good at letting go; they excelled, instead, in collecting one another. There was no such thing as leaving—neither in moves to California nor in death did anyone really get or break away. The dead were not let go; much as their presence was hated, they lived on in the identifications and mannerisms of the living. The survivors simply took them inside and added them to the accumulation of the family legacy. America became the family's self-imposed "Babylonian" captivity.

Bitterness best characterized them—toward Russia, toward America, toward each other, toward their children, toward the future. Their expectation of catastrophe always exceeded and overwhelmed their expectation and attainment of success. The more they acquired, the more they stood to lose—and the more tenaciously they clung to everyone and everything they possessed. They were grateful to their land of opportunity, yet they still felt cheated and deprived. They brought their grievance against history to each new occasion. New rules and roles had little place for their ancient dreams and nightmares.

What did their weighty scholarship and their erstwhile prestige matter? Who here understood their past or was even interested in it? Anybody here could go into business and make a buck. Who cared if one's family had connections to a distant king's court? None of the family's claims on history could be recognized or "cashed in." The family was wealthy—one could almost say "established" once again—but adrift in time. And none on the outside or the inside of the family could put into words, let alone utter, the loss too painful to be remembered and mourned. And even if it could have been remembered, it *dared* not be mourned; for to mourn was to acknowledge loss. To mourn was to betray; it was to "kill" the dead by not keeping them—all of them—alive in oneself.

At last, and pathetically, the "sick role" became the throne upon which the claim to exalted status in America could finally sit and rest. To be sick formed one's own and the family's triumphant vindication. One could at last demand to be treated royally—and others would have to capitulate to the demand, because one was diagnosed as being *officially* sick. One by one, for at least two generations, the family members would find in the sick role exemption from the grueling, humiliating grind of the workaday world.

A host of "real," organic diseases was diagnosed by their physicians. Many retired early from their businesses. Others received disability incomes and disability roles simultaneously. Not that this stopped them from working: some of them could now devote themselves completely and without distraction to their properties and their families (the latter being yet another form of property). Still others, not fortunate enough to be declared as having organic disease, found their way into the sick role via hypochondriasis—and eventual biomedically irreversible disease and death.

The behavior of one whom many in the family described as a "slave-driver" father or grandfather who had demanded that the brood "wait on him hand and foot" could now be legitimately emulated. If one could not be back home in Russia under the protection of an eighteenth century tsar and his village officials, one could at least be a patient under the care of the doctor and receive the guilt-laden devotion of the family. To be sick, to be cared for, and to die in America—this was the best compromise with history one could make. After nearly one hundred years in the United States, it was *still* too painful to sever emotional connections with the Russia the family had once fled in terror.

Family history and its myriad clinical histories, however, are more than what evil tsars, Russian pogromists, and American anti-Semites did to Jews. History is not altogether made or written from the outside in. History is more than the myth of great deeds, great men, and great events as experienced by those upon whom such deeds and events are inflicted. To say that great men (and women) are exponents of their age, or that they have arrived at the right moment in their culture's history, is tantamount to acknowledging that the "great" are at least to some degree the products of the "small." Made for each other, so to speak, they together make what we call "history." This, at least, is the conclusion of such scholars as Abse and Ulman (1977), Binion (1976), deMause (1984), Devereux (1955), Erikson (1958), Gonen (1975), Koenigsberg (1975), La Barre (1972), Stierlin (1976), Volkan (1980), and Volkan and Itzkowitz (1984).

To this family, tsars and *muzhiks* (peasants) were inner presences as much as they were outer realities. Almost agelessly, in this family's mental accounting book, there were good ones and evil ones, inside the family and out. There was the good tsar and the evil one. There was the rabbi-scholar and, a generation or two earlier, the even more saintly one who recounted the Jews' plight before the Russian court. By contrast, there were those whom family standard-bearers contemptuously described as people who "didn't amount to anything." Resentment of the tyranny at the hands of the current family patriarchs could be displaced and projected onto machinations in the distant Kremlin or in the nearby village police.

Inside the family ghetto, it was prohibitively difficult to distinguish between one's protectors and those from whom one required protection. Over many generations, there was desperate and doomed pleading for personal breathing space *within* the family. Devastating as was the status decline at the hands of tsars and police who turned a blind eye to Jews' vulnerabilities, this waning served likewise as rationalization, screen, and focus on which to displace attention from the bitterness and rage sown from childhood experience. One might say that this family—indeed, the wider ethnic-religious group—was dangerously susceptible to recurrent historical traumas of rejection, expulsion, and murder. The outer history—the Gentile history—they suffered and endured was hopelessly and agelessly entangled with the history they also made. Victims of themselves in concert with their circumstances, they ultimately could become victors only in the throes of illness's victory as well.

The unutterable meaning of the family's symptoms and diseases and sick roles lies in the burden of history that the family bore and relentlessly inflicted upon itself. To say that its symptoms and diseases were "symbolic" as well as biomedical entities makes them more, rather than less, real and intelligible. Learning what a family's diseases and symptoms and roles are about can take decades— even generations. The two emigrant generations of my family died out decades ago. The third, "fully American" generation is now entering old age. Not long ago, the family buried one member of this generation. She was my mother. As her life drew to a close, her disease and problem lists were a mile long. They enumerated what all she died with. They could not begin to intimate the family story of what she died from.

There are unmistakable lessons to be garnered from my personal and family story and transposed to that aspect of my life termed "professional": clinical teaching, intern and resident supervision, Balint groups (which discuss difficult physician-patient, physician-physician, and physician-staff relationships, see Scheingold 1988), and direct patient encounters. As should be clear already from earlier chapters, it is a matter of what linguists call "punctuation" to say where "personal" leaves off and the boundary of "professional" begins. Indeed, the very blurring of the boundary can lead to profound insight into other people and to profound distortion of them (such is the dual-edged sword called countertransference). Ultimately, the ability to understand others, to help them clinically or in the classroom, is *always* mediated by one's self.

From my own "case" I have learned somewhat more tolerance for the *ambiguity* and *complexity* and *uncertainty* of physicians' cases (i.e., those cases in which interns, residents, and faculty physicians involve me) and for the selfsame ambiguity and complexity and uncertainty in physicians themselves as these are evoked and played out through the clinical material. I have gained anew a respect for the *timing* of insight (and its lack or lapse), a recognition that neither in myself nor in those whom I teach nor in those with and upon whom physicians practice medicine can such insight and working through be forced or rushed—only facilitated through compassionate, good enough listening. I am reminded that, for patients, families, physicians, and other practitioners alike, the readiness for such insight and renewed integration is greater during painful times of life transition (e.g., pregnancy, birth, adolescence, marriage, divorce, job change, events of personal success or failure, death and other losses).

I have learned somewhat greater humility about the supposed efficacy of scientific—albeit magically used—tools for exhuming family history, family function, and family structure. Because the genogram is one of the discipline-defining (and identity-maintaining) tools of family medicine (Pendagast and Sherman 1977; McGoldrick and Gerson 1985), I have learned to use it as a part of the professional language of the specialty. I have even developed complex genograms of my own multigeneration family of origin—including information about diseases, occupations, migration and settlement, emotional closeness and distance, conflict and alliance—for teaching purposes. I use it as a device with which to collect family data, for the building of rapport with a patient or a physician resident, and for a mental scaffolding constructed "out there" on a piece of paper or a blackboard, safely distant from the patient or intern to begin to discuss vexing problems, a kind of playfully used "transitional object" (Winnicott 1953) that is both "me" and "not me"—a bridge, as it were, to a more internal, unconscious material. Yet for all my experience in using it clinically and didactically, it was of no help to me in this most current understanding of disease, life, and death in my maternal family.

In truth, the family historical material in this chapter came to me, as if I were in some altered state of consciousness, a day or so after the unveiling of my mother's gravestone in September 1986. I was sitting in the living room of my father's apartment, the apartment where I had spent my childhood and adolescence. Suddenly, as if from the outside—although I was certainly conscious that the source was inner—I began to be flooded with fragments of memories, images, and feelings that I had not realized I even "knew" before. I wanted to understand why she had been sick, why she had been sick the ways she had, and why she died. The overwhelming flood was the "answer" (incomplete, since no insight is complete) to my questions.

The lesson I draw from this for clinical teaching and practice is that no clinical tool—genograms, family structural assessments, etc.—can automatically "give" or "elicit" patient (or physician or teacher) insights and resolutions. At most, we can—with compassion, confrontation, and interpretation—stimulate the unconscious, analogous perhaps to the biomedical "prepping" for surgery. But the unending task of understanding oneself, one's family, one's culture, is accomplished by oneself as surgeon and patient both, perhaps in the presence of another who facilitates it or who accompanies oneself on the journey, but it is not done *by* another. Nor is any clinical tool a magical wand to be used ritualistically to achieve insight, change, or resolution. As teachers and clinicians, we can at best set the "stage" or "tone" for another. To the extent that I can tolerate my own ambivalence and temper my own ambitions in seminars, consultations, counseling, and supervision with medical students, interns, residents, and medical faculty, to that degree do I help them to do likewise with patients and their families in clinical practice.

This "case" has given my professional self a greater sense of hope and a deeper sense of limitation and tragedy in any "intervention" with whatever category of person (not those termed "patients" alone). Paradoxically, as I become somewhat liberated from the shackles of my own history by becoming aware of them—or feeling their presence constraining my emotional limbs, so to speak—I become better able to foster such liberation in medical personnel and in patients by finding it less necessary to impose my own shackles upon them.

REFERENCES

Abse, D. W., and R. B. Ulman. 1977. Charismatic political leadership and collective regression. In *Psychopathology and political leadership*, edited by R. S. Robins, 35–52. New Orleans: Tulane University Press.

Binion, R. 1976. *Hitler among the Germans*. New York: Elsevier.

DeMause, L. 1984. *Reagan's America*. New York: Psychohistory Press.

Devereux, G. 1955. Charismatic leadership and crisis. In *Psychoanalysis and the social sciences* edited by G. Roheim, 4:145–57. New York: International Universities Press.

Erikson, E. H. 1958. *Young Man Luther*. New York: Norton.

Feder, S. 1978. Gustav Mahler, dying. *International Review of Psycho-Analysis* 5:125–148.

Gonen, J. Y. 1975. *A psychohistory of Zionism*. New York: Mason/Charter.

Koenigsberg, R. A. 1975. *Hitler's ideology: A study in psychoanalytic sociology*. New York: The Library of Social Science.

La Barre, W. 1972. *The Ghost Dance: The origins of religion*. New York: Dell.

McGoldrick, M., and R. Gerson. 1985. *Genograms in family assessment*. New York: Norton.

Pendagast, E. G., and C. O. Sherman. 1977. A guide to the genogram family systems training. *The Family* 5(1):3–14.

Scheingold, L. 1988. Balint work in England: Lessons for American family medicine. *The Journal of Family Practice* 26(3):315–20.

Stierlin, H. 1976. *Adolf Hitler: A family perspective.* New York: Psychohistory Press.

Volkan, V. D. 1980. Narcissistic personality organization and "reparative" leadership. *The International Journal of Group Psychotherapy* 30(2):131–52.

Volkan, V. D., and N. Itzkowitz. 1984. *The immortal Atatürk: A psychobiography.* Chicago: University of Chicago Press.

Weisman, A. D., and R. K. Kastenbaum. 1968. *The psychological autopsy.* New York: Human Sciences Press.

Winnicott, D. W. 1953. Transitional objects and transitional phenomena. *International Journal of Psycho-Analysis* 34:89–97.

CHAPTER 8

Toward an Integration of Countertransference and Family-of-Origin Perspectives in Medicine

HOWARD F. STEIN

INTRODUCTION

In recent years a considerable literature has developed on the influence of physician (or, more generically, clinician/health-care practitioner) family-of-origin issues on the physician-patient relationship and clinical work itself (Christie-Seely et al. 1984; Crouch 1986; Mengel 1985, 1987; Schwartzman 1986). Mengel, for instance, notes that the out-of-awareness repetition of one's early familial relationships and rules in clinical roles often results in physician ineffectiveness (1987). A parallel literature on the influence of unconscious factors in all aspects of clinical decision making, research, and treatment has developed within the fields of psychoanalysis, psychiatry, and psychoanalytic anthropology (e.g., Davidson 1986; Devereux 1967; Freud 1905, 1923; Katz 1984; Kernberg 1965; Reich 1951; Smith and Stein 1987; Stamm 1987; Stein 1985, 1986a; Stein and Apprey 1985, 1987). The confluence of the countertransference model and the family-of-origin model is explored through a case illustration in which I served as a behavioral science consultant/supervisor with a family medicine resident.

I shall not attempt to review the extensive, even hairsplitting, discussions of countertransference in the literature, but refer the interested reader to the above partial list. Rather, I would summarize it (and, admittedly, oversimplify it as well) by noting the distinction between the "classical" and "totalistic" models of countertransference. According to the classical view, countertransference consists of the antitherapeutic emotional response of the clinician to the patient's own transference. In this view, both responses consist of the "transference" onto current relationships of feelings one had toward persons early in one's life. According to the totalistic view, formulated by Kernberg (1965), countertransference refers to "the total emotional reaction of the psychoanalyst [or clinician of any type] to the patient in the treatment situation" (1965:38). Depending upon the clinician's degree of awareness of and access to his or her own emotions, such countertransference reaction can be equally a source of distortion and a profoundly important technical tool of therapy.

The sense in which I use *countertransference* in this chapter, linking it with *distortions* introduced by out-of-awareness family-of-origin issues, is more the classical view than the totalistic one. I shall argue that both countertransference and family-of-origin distortions of clinical work have the quality and dynamic of "acting out," not in the often construed sense of "poor impulse control" or "willfulness," but rather, in Greenson's words, as "a repetition in action instead of words, memories, and affects" (1967:68). The "language" of clinical distortion is that of action, as a defense against painful remembering and feeling (e.g., Calogeras 1982).

Since there are so many unconscious impediments to such remembering and feeling, the question arises not only *what* (content) a study of one's family of origin can reveal, but *how* (process) one gains access to the very material one is "trying" not to see, hear, or feel. The process of discovery—or recovery—is a key to the hidden material itself. Over the past decade, I have often seen, for instance, in family medicine/family systems training the matter-of-fact, almost mechanical, use and preparation of genograms, whether by physicians with patients or in seminar exercises teaching residents about genograms. Study of family of origin can be used and taught as an exercise that utilizes those same defenses—intellectualization, rationalization, splitting, isolation, etc.—that frequently plague psychoanalysis and psychodynamic psychotherapy! In the case study that follows, I direct the reader to the issue of *how* and *when* emotional and family-of-origin *issues emerge* as much as to the content of the material itself.

Before presenting the case, let me illustrate this issue of emergence with a brief personal example, one that I discuss at length elsewhere (Stein 1988, see chapter 7 of this volume). It was as I was sitting in the living room of my father's apartment—where I had spent my first seventeen years—on the day following the unveiling of my mother's gravestone, nearly a year following her death, that I experienced overwhelming sadness and with it a flood of memories about her, and my, family. These feelings, memories, and family "facts" had been "there" in the sense of dormant information all along, but I had never before integrated these associations as fully as I did then. Here, one might say, a major personal/family *life transition* triggered the emergence of *emotions* that in turn triggered a "train" of associations that made me more fully aware of a deeper level of my *family-of-origin* story.

This oversimplified vignette illustrates a further factor complicating the reconstruction of family-of-origin issues: remembering and piecing together family-of-origin conflicts, patterns, repetitive sequences, roles, rules, secrets, taboos, and the like is never mere cognitive recall. The language of the child and the language of the adult are profoundly different (Ferenczi 1933). Clinically inappropriate, countertherapeutic responses to patients can be viewed as compromise formations or symbols that simultaneously act out unresolved, unconscious family-of-origin issues *and* protect the clinician from feeling or experiencing deeper hurts and more intolerable fantasies (e.g., separation anxiety, rage toward those upon whom one is dependent, etc.). In a book on supervision via the analysis of therapist countertransference, Masterson writes, for instance, that "To the degree to which you have not resolved your own depression (not necessarily an abandonment depression), you will have great difficulty tolerating your patient's depression, because it stimulates your own. It resonates with a lot of the things which you experienced as a child which you have repressed, and it stimulates them and starts tugging on them; they start pushing up, trying to get release" (1983:188).

The following case illustrates how the eruption of countertransference, together with an attempt to understand it, led subsequently to the recovery of family-of-origin issues and their associated deeper feelings.

CASE EXAMPLE

At a patient review conference, Dr. X presented the case of a young woman who had a poorly nourished female infant, diagnosed as failure to thrive. Dr. X looked and talked as though emotionally drained as he presented this case. He had taken steps with Child Welfare to have the female infant removed from the home.

Listening to the presentation, I recalled that Dr. X had recently been instrumental in removing a two and one-half year old male failure-to-thrive child from his mother.

I resolved to visit with Dr. X privately following the conference. I found Dr. X standing in the hallway. I said "This must feel like a hall of mirrors: now not one failure-to-thrive infant, but two, and their families." Dr. X replied, "I'm getting the reputation of being the doctor who takes children out of their homes."

Shortly thereafter, I was met by Dr. X, who said urgently that he wanted to talk with me about a conference presentation he was preparing for noon that day. Dr. X had been ruminating about it a lot, but had not yet sorted out or outlined all that he wanted to say. We entered the conference room and did a "dance" of where to sit; Dr. X was very uneasy. He had already voluntarily put a thorough three-generation genogram on the magic-marker board and sat with several pages of notes. The genogram was that of Ms. W, whose two and one-half year old son, Arnold, he had months earlier diagnosed as failure to thrive. Dr. X. had initiated removing Arnold from Ms. W's care. He asked me to help him to go back and correctly reconstruct this previous case that he was having difficulty remembering because it had been so emotional for him.

My familiarity with this case, and with the physician's distress about its outcome, had begun at a patient review conference months earlier. Dr. X's patient, Arnold, was initially presented as an interesting biomedical diagnostic problem. Born three months premature, he had hydrocephalus and lagged in his growth curve. Six months earlier, his mother, Ms. W, a twenty-three year old white, unmarried woman with one other child, had brought him to another clinic for vomiting, fever, lethargy, and "spells." Dr. X saw him first three months later, and diagnosed him as having failure to thrive.

Two months following the initial visit, the baby was hospitalized, and following discharge the mother brought him four or five times to the emergency room during the subsequent two months, due to the child's vomiting and lethargy. The child seemed to have a pattern of improving eating and weight gain while in the hospital, and lethargy, vomiting, fever of 102 degrees F., and tantrums while back at home. A major medical work-up at a distant urban medical center revealed no biomedical causes for this pattern. The physician described poor mother-child bonding, and began the process of seeking foster-care through Child Welfare to have the child removed from the home. Ms. W was divorced and pregnant by her current boyfriend. Her own mother and grandmother (in their forties and sixties respectively) appealed to Dr. X to have the baby given to the grandmother's care, rather than to Child Welfare.

At the patient-review conference noted above, the resident and faculty pursued the diagnostic enigma. To the pattern of symptoms were now added bloating, abdominal distention, and frequent burping. Among the diseases considered in the differential diagnosis were Addison's disease, giardia, seizure disorders (to be ruled out by electroencephalogram), and renal acidosis. The resident said that he had begun the case months ago thinking that the baby's problems were primarily constitutional, exacerbated perhaps by a bad home situation. The conclusion of this conference was that the resident should get a pediatrics consult on the case. I had commented at the time of this case presentation that, in addition to the support the infant needed, it sounded as if the mother and her family could use some counseling as well.

Later that afternoon Dr. X had said urgently, "I gotta talk with you." At the beginning of our discussion, Dr. X's pupils had been widely dilated, his voice had had a slight quiver, he was breathing hard, and his eyes had seemed to be slightly tearful. In response to Child Welfare personnel's questioning on the phone, he had expressed willingness to testify in court that he believed Ms. W was an unfit mother, but he did not know what was said to her when they had gone to pick up the toddler. Earlier that afternoon he had learned that Ms. W had come in to the clinic for her medical records and had contacted an attorney to reclaim Arnold from Child Welfare. Although Dr. X had felt confident in his medical judgment, he dreaded the prospect of long legal proceedings. He was in panic.

I had asked Dr. X about his previous communication with Ms W. He had said that he had explained things over and over again medically to her, but that he just had not been able to bring himself to say to her: "You're a lousy mother. You don't love your child." Dr. X had said, "When I'm talking with a patient, I try to keep the discussion to medical things, like the baby isn't getting enough nutrition, that it's failing to thrive. My mistake is to keep the psycho-social things out and not to deal with them with the mother."

I had asked him if he had an idea of why it was so difficult for him to bring up things that might provoke conflict. His eyes had widened even further, and his voice had quivered: "The way I was raised, you never spoke up. If you didn't like something, you kept quiet. Because if you did speak up, say you didn't like something, you got hit upside your head. You learned to keep things inside, because you knew the consequences if you didn't." He did not appear to be merely remembering a remote event; he was reliving it. I had asked him to clarify, and it was clear that he had meant getting slapped, beaten, for speaking his mind. We hadn't discussed who had administered the physical punishment in Dr. X's own family of origin, but it had been clear to us both that Dr. X was transferring his early situation to the present one, and thus had been unable to talk candidly with Ms. W. I had urged Dr. X to contact Child Welfare and to find out their assessment of the home situation of Ms. W, so that he could know and respond to the real current situation and not only act upon his inner dread.

We sat in the conference room looking at the genogram that Dr. X had drawn for Ms. W and her family. I gently questioned where Dr. X "fit" into the family diagram, since Dr. X had written "me" with arrows beneath Ms. W and her children. Dr. X would talk about himself and his family, then switch back to Ms. W's family, using the genogram to distance himself. He said that Ms. W's family had characterized itself as close-knit and supportive, yet at the delivery of her third infant, only her boyfriend had been present. Her only additional visitor to the hospital had been her ex-husband's mother. Dr. X questioned whether this family's closeness was in word only rather than in deed.

Dr. X reflected that Ms. W seemed to be off of drugs (although she continued to smoke marijuana, which she did not consider to be a "drug") since the recent birth of her third child, a daughter. With her boyfriend, over these past months, she had somewhat separated herself from her considerably alcoholic/drug-prone family. Dr. X was still worried about Arnold's future, especially since Arnold continued to have lethargy–vomiting spells every eight to ten days at the home of the foster parents, just as he had had at his natal home. Dr. X was puzzled about how much the failure to thrive was psychosocial and how much medical. He said that he had difficulty emotionally reliving and accurately remembering what he had *felt* like when he had learned that Ms. W was in contact with a lawyer regarding custody of Arnold. He asked me to help assist him in doing so, since he wanted to be able to discuss this at his conference presentation.

Dr. X began to talk about his fear of "being put on the stand" and seeing Ms. W and the judge "pronouncing judgment over me." He identified as "panic" his earlier frightening feeling upon hearing of

Mrs. W's phone call that she was coming to take her medical chart to a lawyer. With some prompting, Dr. X cautiously offered further associations about his own family of origin.

> When I was little and I wanted to say anything, I had better be right. My mom and dad would ask me something, and when I answered the question, I'd better come up with the right answer or they'd hit me upside the face. [I asked him to clarify the phrase "upside the face." Dr. X continued,] I'd get beaten and sometimes I'd be hit on the face. You learned never to speak just glibly, 'cause the consequences were great. You learned to watch yourself and keep your mouth shut unless you were sure of yourself.
>
> With Arnold, I started out thinking that his failure to thrive was psychosocial in origin, but since then I've become less sure; it's true that he was given a thorough work-up in the hospital which produced nothing. Just before he went there he went through one of his episodes, and sure enough when he was there he was just normal—and as soon as he returned home ten days later he started getting lethargic and nauseous! I've started to think lately that I should have given more credence to the medical side of things. Maybe I could have come up with the right answer that way. I could just see Ms. W, the judge, and the jury looking at me and saying "Why didn't you get more aggressive with the medical stuff?" I think that's why I have this medical/psychosocial split. I started thinking initially that I could come up with the right answers with psychosocial stuff, but then I got scared—thinking about being up there on the stand. It was either/or, and the psychosocial had let me down. It was frightening, because I was expected to come up with the right answers or else, Whomp upside the head.

I interpreted, "Just like when you were small." He gave a "yeh" of recognition.

I said, "With these kids, you're going through your pain all over again, feeling like the child at the hands of unreliable parents." Dr. X replied urgently, poignantly: "You want them to have it better than you had when you were their age. I feel myself identifying with these kids. What can they do to help themselves? I feel for them. I want to do right by them. But then I worry about the parents or grandparents saying in court 'What do you mean I don't love my child?'" I brought up Dr. X's possible wish to punish the parents, as he wished to get back at his own parents for what they did to him: "That's there. I don't understand how a parent could act the way they do." I urged him to become more conscious of and control the wish to punish them, since it could interfere with his clinical judgment. I redirected him temporarily back to that aspect of himself that he had projectively identified with in these neglected children: i.e., the harrowing feeling he has that *he* was unloved by *his* parents.

I said to Dr. X, "Cases like this are your 'Achilles heel'; different physicians are vulnerable to different kinds of cases or problems." He concurred, "When I agonize about this case in conference, I can see that with other residents it's no big thing. Other kinds of cases bother them. I'm the one who's really bent out of shape by this case, where there's neglect or abuse." Dr. X began to distinguish between the child's reality and his own fantasy, to assess realistically the child's home situation as separate from his projection/rescue fantasy born of his own miserable childhood. Dr. X began to realize that one of the major functions (mental/emotional functions) of the biomedical model and of medical decision making was to provide *him* the authority and certainty so that he would not be wrong in his answers and thereby would avoid being put in the situation of helplessness at the hands of medical faculty and colleagues, successors to his parents.

The current case resembled and evoked the past for Dr. X. Momentarily feeling his sense of vulnerability, I identified with him and offered the interpretation that perhaps Dr. X felt now like an endangered Arnold at the hands of his family. Dr. X stood up, and walked over to the board, his eyes riveted on the genogram. He said: "There's more here than meets the eye. When I was two or three, my parents divorced. My dad, whom I can't remember, just up and left. He left for another woman, leaving my mom high and dry to take care of everything. I had two sisters. She had to take all the responsibility. A year or so later, she married. He says he loves me, that he's glad we're in the family, and all that. But I've often wondered whether that's just what he thinks we'd like to hear. I don't know what he really thinks and feels about me, whether he ever really wanted me." I pointed out the parallel between this and Ms. W's family's official myth of closeness and actual abandonment or at least vacillation. Dr. X tearfully recognized the parallel. Interestingly, during the subsequent case conference presentation, he did not set himself up to repeat the family dynamic in which he was the helpless child and the other participants were dangerous, critical, brutal parents.

Commenting on the case, Johanna Shapiro notes "how the resident in question was almost obsessive in his identification of 'failure-to-thrive' kids, as though he might, with sufficient diligence, rescue the entire universe of deprived children (and perhaps nurture himself in the process)" (personal communication, 30 November

1987). In its psychological aim, as distinct from its specific content, the physician's *reparative* behavior plays out a universal fantasy: to "repair" our very selves and our imperfect childhoods even as we relive and restage our rawest vulnerabilities.

DISCUSSION AND CONCLUSION

Here I wish to consider several meanings of the case just summarized. I hope to demonstrate that, far from being limited to the individual physician's countertransference and family of origin, the case reverberates as well with psychosocial issues prevalent throughout the institution of medicine and the wider American culture. To begin with, the case illustrates the point that *what* one remembers (content) is closely related to *how* one remembers and *when* one remembers. Freud wrote that "The repressed retains its upward urge, its effort to force its way to consciousness" (1939:95). Among the three conditions under which the repressed material returns to consciousness is "if at any time in recent experience impressions or experiences occur which resemble the repressed so closely that they are able to awaken it. In this case the recent experience is reinforced by the latent energy of the repressed, and the repressed comes into operation behind the recent experience with its help" (1939:95). Thus, the *timing* of the remembering is part of the memory, part of the accessibility to the reconstruction itself.

How the recollection and reconstruction occurred in this case was via the resident's panic reaction, together with consultations in which he was not punished for his "error" of imperfection, enabling his own exploration of emotion-laden family-of-origin issues. A degree of mutual *identification* between Dr. X and me, as behaviorial science consultant, facilitated the transition from resident countertransference to reliving and integrating terrifying family-of-origin experiences into his awareness. His uncovering and recovering of deep-seated, unconscious, family-of-origin issues was mediated by a *relationship in the present* that facilitated greater integration rather than compelling further repression and splitting of traumatic family-of-origin experiences and their associated affects (e.g., rage, terror, intense separation anxiety, helplessness). The sequence of the recovery of family-of-origin issues is schematically represented in figure 8.1.

The physician with whom I consulted could be said to be symptomatic in at least two senses: (1) what might be regarded as the "objective" fact of the return of the repressed, followed by a panic

During patient encounters with Arnold and his mother, awakening of physician's unresolved family-of-origin issues of abandonment and neglect; identification with Arnold.

Psychosocial diagnosis of Arnold's failure to thrive, but strictly biomedical exploration and communication with Ms. W about this diagnosis. Inability to communicate with Ms. W about psychosocial issues in Arnold's failure to thrive.

T   Rescue action to remove Arnold from "bad" family.

I   Ms. W comes to clinic for Arnold's file; Dr. X fears that
M   he is wrong, that the psychosocial diagnosis is the
E   source of being wrong, and that he will be punished by
      Ms. W and the court.

S   Panic . . . return of the repressed . . . dread of "being
E   put on the stand" and seeing the patient's mother
Q   and judge "pronounce judgment over me" (a con-
U   temporary replay of what we later discover to be his
E   own fear of punishment at the hands of his parents
N   when he was small).
C   Reawakening of savagely punitive conscience, reexperi-
E   ence helplessness in family of origin, expectation of
      beatings.

Consultant (HFS) does not criticize or punish him for his "errors," but explores their meaning with him.

Physician begins to reconstruct family-of-origin traumatic situations and to reexperience their associated emotions (rage, helplessness, separation anxiety), working through rather than avoiding them.

Integration of painful emotions and memories into consciousness; gradual separation of core fantasy (fear of recurrent punishment and abandonment, based on family-of-origin situation and associated affects) from reality of the patient and family (current medical situation).

Diminished need to use biomedicine defensively and to disparage psychosocial theory and methods; increased insight into the personal significance for him of failure to thrive/abused children, diminution of projection of his original situation onto them, increase in ability to evaluate current cases individually.

Figure 8.1   Sequence of recovery of family-of-origin issues

reaction; (2) the fact that the physician felt himself to have a problem and asked my assistance in its solution (i.e., as if to say "I have a
symptom"). I would argue that, beyond being temporarily symptomatic "himself," he is also symptomatic of a familial, medical
cultural, and wider cultural organization or system that place such a
premium on being certain and always right. His failure of personal
defenses likewise illumines the professional defensive organization
of medicine. Professional training in medicine and patient care
constitute *new contexts in which the old unconscious and family-of-origin
issues are replayed with new role partners* (see also Schwartzman 1986).
This physician had *consciously* chosen a medical career in part as a
way of escaping his early abusive environment. *Unconsciously,* however, having identified with it, he replicated it, albeit expressing his
symptom in a socially acceptable and prestigious form (Devereux
1980:94–100).

I have thus far attempted to explicate the relationship between
countertransference and family-of-origin issues, and to understand
the process whereby one gains access to unconscious feelings, memories, roles, and so forth that are formidably well defended. The
interpretation offered suggests that the dichotomy between unconscious issues and family-of-origin issues is likely a spurious one,
since the two are different facets of the same phenomenon. The
issue of "what happened," and the intrapsychic elaboration of or
meaning of "what happened," are equally important (Masterson
1985:170–71; Terry 1984). In the above case, the physician's countertransference to the case served as a point of departure for our
exploration of this family-of-origin dynamics and their personal
significance for him.

Beyond the individual case that links individual unconscious and
family systems dynamics, this case sheds light on a number of issues
of social theory and clinical practice beyond the case itself. Among
these are: What is the scope or extent of the mental dynamics that
kept the resident's attitudinal/value/behavioral set going this long
(Stein 1984a, 1986b)? What is the articulation or "fit" between
culture and personality dynamics? How does culture and institutional (e.g., occupational, professional) setting replay or restage
(Binion 1981) early recurrent trauma, conflict, and defenses against
them? How does cultural and institutional continuity occur (e.g.,
the process via the affirmation of the defenses), and how does culture change at a deep level occur (e.g., the process of emotional/
intellectual understanding of what the defenses were fending off)?

How and when do individual, personal countertransference responses patterns become institutionally mobilized (normalized, reinforced, put to use) and culturally reaffirmed—both to the individual (physician) and to the wider group?

Can shared unconscious conflict (i.e., present not only idiosyncratically in this physician, but throughout biomedicine and more widely throughout the culture) be bound and symbolized through shared defenses against it (i.e., in the form of shared representations and rituals)? One of the mental functions of the culturally elaborated "medical model" is for the physician (and other health-care personnel as well) to "have the right answers" to give to authority figures (successors and representatives of parents) and in turn to function as authority figures. At a deeper level, this averts punishment, humiliation, and threat of abandonment, in order to stave off rage and depression over possible abandonment (see Katz 1984; Stein 1985; Stein and Apprey 1985). This statement characterizes both the individual resident's situation *and* the rather typical dynamics of medical education and practice.

Normative American medical cultural values and attitudes—normative in the dual sense of prescriptions *for* behavior and descriptions *of* widespread behavior—consist of control, the quest for completeness, mastery, omnipotence, omniscience, the ability to cure or "fix" virtually any problem, certainty, intolerance of ambiguity, need to have "the answer" and the expectation that everything does have a discrete answer, the equation of inability to cure with personal failure or patient's moral inadequacy, and/or the reduction of complexity to simplicity (doctrine of specific etiology extended to all aspects of explanation and care). Now, these widespread values and attitudes are inculcated in medical school, internship, residency, and later during practice through peer pressure, identificatory processes (e.g., identification with the aggressor), the rote learning of voluminous data, the pedagogical technique of "pimping," the dread of being "gooned" and thereby publicly humiliated by a superior, and the combination of long hours "on call" with sleep deprivation. The rigor of medical education assures for most in the elder and successor generation the *continuity* of repetition of intrusive—if not persecutory—family-of-origin style, now reenacted in the teaching status and role hierarchy (e.g., teacher/student, intern/student, resident/intern, physician/nurse).

The clinical authoritarian style is further reaffirmed and evoked by many patients who—even as they are in recent decades demanding greater autonomy and equality in the clinical relationship—demand and expect a "magical" cure for all of life's afflictions. Some threaten malpractice litigation if a less than perfect medical solution occurs. Through displacement and projection, physicians repeatedly "relive" their earlier developmental traumas and conflicts as evoked by parallel emotional situations in their medical training and practice settings (e.g., patients' transference). Johanna Shapiro comments that the above case expresses "widespread, culturally bound repressions and defenses, which . . . characterize the medical education system and to a large degree our society in general. Coming from the family he did, this poor resident must have felt right at home training to be a doctor, where you get 'whomped upside the head'" (personal communication, 30 November 1987). Medical training is unconsciously designed to help physicians shore up their defenses against these old and recurrent threats by first assaulting them and then offering protection against these induced threats.

Sadly, this has the characteristic of a "protection racket" (see Stein 1984b) in which protectors first endanger those whom they will offer protection. Shared traumas and conflicts are endlessly repeated, and institutional/professional defenses against them are offered to each generation of professional initiates. Among such defenses are the need for certainty and the belief that it can be found, and the need to be right and the belief that through adherence to clinical orthodoxies one can be assured of being right. Through this ritual process, succeeding generations are taught what to remember and what to forget—thereby reaffirming in the generations of clinical elders their own distinction between what can and what cannot be tolerated to enter clinical consciousness.

What, then, are the boundaries of the resident's symptoms (Stein 1984a)? Clearly, his panic reaction is pathognomonic. But what of his erstwhile defensive organization, one that is, in turn, at least to a degree, shared with and shaped by the institution of biomedicine and the culture it serves? Depending upon one's vantage point, is the physician not a part of the group symptomatology and the group not part of his "individual" symptoms? From the case presented, the physician was temporarily symptomatic in the more conventional sense that he acknowledged, at some level at least, that he had and was part of the problem; that, at least momentarily, his defenses, and their institutional counterparts, had failed him. The case study identified (1) the emotional correspondence between the current clinical situation and his early family-of-origin situation; (2)

the failure of his personal defenses, unleashing; (3) the return of the repressed, and with it, panic.

However, to these surely must be added the *induced* anxiety-and-defense organization of the medical training and practice setting, a situation that supersedes even as it recapitulates his prior family experience. Ego-syntonic character organization can be regarded as symptomatic even though the individual and his/her "reference" group use them as their measure of sanity, reality, normality, legality, and coherence (Freud 1927; La Barre 1972; Devereux 1980). C. R. Badcock, for instance, argues that *"from the point of view of latent content, there is no way of distinguishing between individual psychopathology and its collective equivalents, such as religion"* (1980:240, emphasis in original). He continues that "Those who in recent years have criticized the notion of mental illness as being an arbitrary category of social definition have entirely missed the point. It is not madness, but sanity which is the arbitrary social category, as is proved by the fact that paranoid delusions, like anti-Semitism, can be regarded as perfectly sane if enough of the population believes in them" (1980:241).

In the above case, the resident's symptoms are his failure of defense, while medicine's and the wider culture's symptoms are the defenses—together with the need for them—themselves. The resident's panic *manifests* those types of core issues that are kept *latent* by the "success" of defense in most others. Devereux astutely writes that "It is simply not enough to call socially acceptable behavior 'sublimation' and socially unacceptable behavior 'symptom.' Yet many 'experts' routinely reason in these terms. Even some psychoanalysts believe that they have helped the patient to sublimate his conflict when all they have done is to replace a socially unacceptable symptom or misevaluation with a socially acceptable one without bringing the patient one inch closer to that culturally undistorted *reality acceptance* that is the touchstone of sanity" (1980:94). It is ironic, if not paradoxical, that the very collapse of the personal/professional defenses in this physician, and his willingness to discuss what was erupting in his mind, helped him to be a more compassionate and less driven physician than colleagues who might be regarded as more culturally "normal."

In this context, for countertransference and family-of-origin issues to enter at all into biomedical training is indeed revolutionary. We who would further this truly revolutionary integration of what has been heretofore banished and repressed from clinical consciousness would better serve the cause of such integration by avoiding the lure of yet another either/or intellectual and clinical polarization: that between the unconscious and family-of-origin influences upon clinical practice.

REFERENCES

Badcock, C. R. 1980. *The psychoanalysis of culture.* Oxford: Basil Blackwell.

Binion, R. 1981. *Soundings: Psychohistorical and psycholiterary.* New York: Psychohistory Press.

Calogeras, R. C. 1982. Sleepwalking and the traumatic experience. *International Journal of Psychoanalysis* 63:483–89.

Christie-Seely, J., R. Fernandez, G. Paradis, Y. Talbot, and R. Turcotte. 1984. The physician's family. In *Working with the family in primary care: A systems approach to health and illness,* edited by J. Christie-Seely, 524–46. New York: Praeger.

Crouch, M. 1986. Working with one's own family: Another path for professional development. *Family Medicine* 18:93–98.

Davidson, R. H. 1986. Transference and countertransference phenomena: The problem of the observer in the behavioral sciences. *Journal of Psychoanalytic Anthropology* 9(3):269–83.

Devereux, G. 1967. *From anxiety to method in the behavioral sciences.* The Hague: Mouton.

———. 1980. *Basic problems of ethno-psychiatry,* translated by B. M. Gulati and G. Devereux. Chicago: University of Chicago Press.

Ferenczi, S. 1933. Confusion of tongues between adults and the child. *International Journal of Psycho-Analysis* 30:225–30.

Freud, S. 1905. Jokes and their relation to the unconscious. In *The standard edition of the complete psychological works of Sigmund Freud (SE)* 8, translated by J. Strachey, 3–236. London: Hogarth Press, 1960.

———. 1923. The ego and the id. *SE* 19, translated by J. Strachey, 3–66. London: Hogarth Press, 1961.

———. 1927. The future of an illusion. *SE* 21, translated by J. Strachey, 5–56. London: Hogarth Press, 1961.

———. 1939. Moses and monotheism. *SE* 23, translated by J. Strachey, 7–137. London: Hogarth Press, 1964.

Greenson, R. R. 1967. *The technique and practice of psychoanalysis.* New York: International Universities Press.

Katz, J. 1984. *The silent world of doctor and patient.* New York: Free Press/Macmillan.

Kernberg, O. F. 1965. Notes on countertransference. *Journal of the American Psychoanalytic Association* 13:38–56.

La Barre, W. 1972. *The ghost dance: The origins of religion.* New York: Dell.

Masterson, J. F. 1983. *Countertransference and psychotherapeutic technique: Teaching seminars on psychotherapy of the borderline adult.* New York: Brunner/Mazel.

———. 1985. *The real self: A developmental, self, and object relations approach.* New York: Brunner/Mazel.

Mengel, M. B. 1985. Collaboration with family therapists: Dealing with physician's family of origin issues. *Working Together* 1:10–11.

————. 1987. Physician ineffectiveness due to family-of-origin issues. *Family Systems Medicine* 5(2):176–90.

Reich, A. 1951. On counter-transference. *International Journal of Psychoanalysis* 32:25–31.

Schwartzman, J. 1986. The natural history of a drug treatment system. *Family Systems Medicine* 4(4):344–57.

Shapiro, J. 1987. Personal communication, 30 November.

Smith, R. C., and H. F. Stein. 1987. A topographical model of clinical decision making and interviewing. *Family Medicine* 19(5):361–63.

Stamm, I. 1987. Countertransference in hospital treatment: Basic concepts and paradigms. Number 2 of a series of occasional papers from The Menninger Foundation. Topeka, Kan.: Menninger Foundation.

Stein, H. F. 1984a. The boundary of the symptom: *Whose* death and dying? *Family Systems Medicine* 2(2):188–94.

————. 1984b. A note on patron-client theory. *Ethos* 12(1):30–36.

————. 1985. *The psychodynamics of medical practice: Unconscious factors in patient care.* Berkeley and Los Angeles: University of California Press.

————. 1986a. "Sick people" and "trolls": A contribution to the understanding of the dynamics of physician explanatory models. *Culture, Medicine and Psychiatry* 10:221–29.

————. 1986b. Social role and unconscious complementarity," *The Journal of Psychoanalytic Anthropology* 9(3):235–68.

————. 1988. Family diseases and family history. *Family Medicine* 20(1):13–15.

Stein, H. F., and M. Apprey. 1985. *Context and dynamics in clinical knowledge,* vol. 1 of the Series in Ethnicity, Medicine, and Psychoanalysis. Charlottesville: University Press of Virginia.

————. 1987. *From metaphor to meaning: Papers in psychoanalytic anthropology,* vol. 2 of the Series in Ethnicity, Medicine, and Psychoanalysis. Charlottesville: University Press of Virginia.

Terry, J. 1984. The damaging effects of the "survivor syndrome." In *Psychoanalytic reflections on the holocaust: Selected essays,* edited by S. A. Luel and P. Marcus, 135–48. New York: Holocaust Awareness Institute, Center for Judaic Studies, University of Denver, and KTAV Publishing House.

CHAPTER 9

Leading by Following: The Ethnographic Study of One's Family as a Tool of Patient Care

HOWARD F. STEIN AND J. MICHAEL PONTIOUS

INTRODUCTION

This chapter illustrates the use of an ethnographic training model in the teaching of behavioral sciences in family medicine and in other clinical specialties. The ethnographic model (Stein 1982b) helps the practitioner-trainee gain access simultaneously to his or her own story and to that of the patient. This model consists of an open-ended, descriptive, long-term, participant-observational, context-dependent approach that gives the resident a feel for families and wider social systems. It helps the resident to make systematic inquiry into the social field in which patient *and* physician move. In this model, the behavioral scientist–family medicine resident relationship (and likewise the colleagueal relationship between behavioral scientists and physician-faculty) is based more on the seemingly paradoxical technique of "leading by following" the resident's leads, interests, and questions than by strict adherence to currently conventional family-data-eliciting and pedagogical instruments (e.g., the genogram [Pendagast and Sherman 1977] the Kvebaek family sculpture [Cromwell, Fournier, and Kvebaek 1980], family functioning inventories [Olson et al. 1982]). Rather, these cultural teaching tools (that is, those widely adopted in resident socialization toward working with the family in contemporary American medicine) are used as points of departure.

We have found that contextual "systems thinking" by residents is enhanced when the behavioral science teacher takes an interest in the family medicine resident's own metaphors and contexts, especially as these are evoked by "difficult" or "interesting" clinical cases, the group dynamics of medical conferences, medical/administrative staff conflicts, and personal or family problems brought by the resident to the behavioral science consultant for discussion. Elsewhere Stein (1985a; Stein and Apprey 1985) has discussed in detail the uses and limits of the analysis of countertransference as a physician training tool. The ethnographic approach here proposed is less a conscious teaching strategy than it is a way of viewing the clinical teaching relationship, one that involves taking a personal interest in the resident's lived reality as we endeavor to teach the resident to take into account that of the patient. It is an approach that begins with an inquiry and acknowledgment of the breadth and depth of the resident's (and all physicians') world and leads the resident to a similar acknowledgment and interest in the world in which the patient moves.

While in family medicine there is an official ideology of the need to teach "systems thinking" and "systems intervention," how we ought to go about teaching about family systems, larger social systems (e.g., the health care system, judicial and legislative institutions, culture), and the relationship all these have to health, illness, and treatment remains a lively question. The culture of American medicine and medical education has long been rife with such dichotomous distinctions as those between "real medicine" or "real (organic) disease" and "social" or "family" contexts; between "hard" and "soft" science and interventions (the former associated with such terms as biomedical, active, procedure, aggressive; the latter, associated with such terms as behavioral science, counseling, talking, passive); between being a "doctor" and being a "therapist" or "counselor." Context and systems teaching are heir to the second, somewhat devalued, member(s) of each of these cultural pairs. While we might wish to teach systems thinking, how do we give residents access to this culturally new and often disparaged style of thinking? This question directs our further attention not only to how we might teach but to how medical students and residents might best learn. In this paper we argue that the issue of how residents learn about systems is inextricable from the content of systems thinking we wish to impart.

The point of departure of what we are calling the ethnographic approach to clinical training is that we teach context by learning, respecting, and working within the resident's own context, rather than by introducing context as something foreign. In this framework, the clinical teacher is not only interested in observing the patient and family but in observing the resident (and oneself) within the wider system that includes patient and family. It is our experience that only the clinical teacher who honors the world the medical student and resident inhabits will be likewise respected, admitted to the student's and resident's more personal world, and thereafter permitted to teach—which is to say, introduce change—within it. The teacher who honors the *culture of medicine* will more readily be allowed to teach about family and wider systems with a breadth and depth that will not be as accessible to the teacher who intrusively seeks to teach about "the family."

Moreover, one's participation as teacher or clinician is part of any system under study or clinical treatment. The physician's subjectivity, while officially disavowed, is nonetheless present (Stein 1982c, 1983b, 1985a; Stein and Apprey 1985). As Alexander profoundly noted some years ago: "participation in a circumstance is always a form of intervention" (1979:64). It is important for the clinical teacher and resident alike to come to know precisely how they participate in the many systems of patient and staff (Schwartzman et al. 1984; Schwartzman 1985).

Physicians bring their experiences in their own families of origin and current families into the clinical encounter, experiences that inadvertently color, if not structure, the physician's perception, expectations, interpretation, interventions, and assumptions about the outcome of that encounter. The physician's own personality and family structure are often unseen intervening variables that mediate clinical relationships. An ethnographic approach includes the investigator within the investigation itself. It reveals that "the process of assessment [is] itself an intervention" (Alexander 1979:89), not simply prefatory to officially punctuated intervention. A greater understanding of the process called "clinical judgment," together with an improvement in that process, can be expected to follow the adoption of an ethnographic approach.

In the ethnographic style of clinical teaching, one seizes the teaching moment (Stein 1983c) and context through which a subject is most learnable. At the same time, this approach allows the observer to select areas for observation that do not generate great anxiety and thereby resistance to the topic. In other words, the best teaching strategy is to lead by following the resident's/ student's lead. One can best teach when and where another is most ready to learn, an approach that especially commends itself to the relatively taboo topic of subjectivity in medicine.

For instance, as reported elsewhere (Stein 1983c), the creative systems teacher can utilize the frequent visits and presentations to teaching clinics/hospitals by pharmaceutical agents as occasions on which to make timely and apt comments about the physician-patient-family relationship with respect to the prescribing and taking of medication. Impromptu case consultations sought by residents or faculty physicians—often at the end of a busy clinic day or unexpectedly at a faculty meeting—are likewise serendipitous, unrehearsable occasions where some of the best and most eager teaching and learning takes place. When a resident or faculty physician feels thwarted by a particularly "difficult" patient, we tactfully inquire into whether the resident or faculty colleague might have faced a parallel difficult situation in his or her family of origin or current family. This, in turn, is often an opportune time to utilize the genogram, for at such moments the resident may become at last persuaded of its utility.

In this use, the genogram serves as a quasi-therapeutic exercise (therapeutic in its dynamics and its outcome, but not in its labeling by the teacher). It helps the resident to discover how the internalized family past is a potent force in his or her professional life. Further, it helps the resident to be more attentive to and accepting of such forces in the lives of his or her patients. Finally, it helps to affect a greater self-differentiation between the physician, the physician's family, the patient, and the patient's family (an approach somewhat similar to that of Murray Bowen [1978]).

Yet another contextual approach with a "difficult" patient involves the behavioral scientist, and occasionally the resident or faculty physician in soliciting additional information about the patient's mood, attitude, etc., from receptionists (who see patients and are often told crucial clinical data by them, and who are valuable yet relatively underutilized health care personnel), medical assistants, nurses, secretaries, and personnel in the business office. Although the behavioral scientist coauthor has formally been consultant to two residency training programs, he has unofficially transformed the role into consultant to the entire clinic at each of the two rural sites. Often only by working closely with the entire "clinic family" can he recommend a patient- or family-intervention to a member of the resident subgroup. It is only through long hours of availability that teaching moments arise and can come to fruition.

A NOTE ON METHODOLOGY

Methodologically, an ethnographic framework for the clinical understanding of any symptom, and therefore for recommending or planning clinical intervention (Stein 1982b, 1983a; Stein and Grant 1986), involves a dual assessment. The first assessment points toward the official focus of clinical concern: the patient, the patient's family, the patient's community and culture, for the purpose of determining pertinent values, expectations, attitudes, and beliefs as they relate to health perceptions and actions. The second points toward the clinician, his/her own family, the clinician's community and culture, the professional culture of medicine, and the wide assortment of other institutional cultures that impinge on patient care (Schwartzman et al. 1984), to determine equally pertinent values, expectations, attitudes, and beliefs as they influence the health care professional and profession's perceptions and actions. An ethnographic understanding of clinical decision making and clinical action would consist of an effort to comprehend the confluence or interplay of these two worlds.

The ethnographic method, which has been the foundation for anthropological fieldwork since early in the twentieth century, is contextual and open-ended. For, in looking, one never knows quite what to look for, and can therefore discover what had been overlooked. The nature and scope of the system must always remain an open-ended question. Moreover, the meaning of any social system for its participants is an intrinsic part of that system, and likewise unconscious process is part of that context. Systematic inquiry based on participant observation and open-ended interviews within a group leads to the uncovering of patterns and levels of meanings and relationships that are often not discernable by standard cultural techniques of data collection. One has a sense for the pattern (whether sequentially over time or repeated over space) when one has a déjà vu feeling about new observations, when new data have the quality of redundancy, and when one is able to begin to predict the flow of events. The ethnographic method, therefore, permits an investigator or clinician to grasp the breadth, complexity, and depth of symptom formation, persistence, and treatment.

Now, at its most sound, the ethnographic method is as much concerned with *how* and *why* we observe as with *what* we observe, for the former heavily influence the latter. We observe through the eyes of our internalized family and culture, seeing with them, so to speak, wherever we go. The ethnographic approach advanced here is a relatively emotionally safe, quasi-therapeutic forum with which to explore subjective factors in clinical judgment, for it directs the student's and resident's focus of attention (initially at least) in the direction both consonant with the direction of medical investigation

and most personally comfortable: that is, *outward*. By taking a naturalistic, as opposed to a prescriptive, approach to family decision
making over issues of health and illness—that is, by inquiring into
the process and logic of that decision making in one's own family
rather than assuming what that logic and outcome in health action
should be—we are doing family ethnography of health and illness
with the student or resident. The goal is never "instant depth"
(which is both unethical and technically misguided), but to begin
with emotionally neutral material and take the student or resident's
lead. By adopting the paradoxical principle of leading by following,
one invariably is led to emotionally valent issues in the student or
resident's own family functioning (Stein and Apprey 1985).

Through immersion in a family or group over long periods of
time, often on its home ground, one learns how that system and its
many subsystems are organized (Geertz 1973; La Barre 1978; Spiro
1982:xv; Stein 1982b, 1983a), and therefore how one might best
intervene medically in it, together with a heightened awareness of
constraints upon such intervention. Through participant observation, in-depth interviewing, and similar open-ended approaches
that minimally structure informants' or patient's responses (e.g.,
often achievable through family medicine's ideal of continuity of
care), the physician or researcher is able to achieve what Geertz calls
a "thick description" (Geertz 1973) of peoples' actual lives and
therefore of the meanings and relationships that underlie health-
related decision making and sickness behavior. In a paper on primary care theory and research, Kleinman advocates the ethnographic method as a means of eliciting meanings associated with
illness and treatment.

> Qualitative description, taken together with various quantitative mea-
> sures, can be a standardized research method for assessing validity. It is
> especially valuable in studying social and cultural significance, e.g.,
> illness beliefs, interaction norms, social gain, ethnic help seeking, and
> treatment responses, and it is the appropriate method to describe the
> work of doctoring. . . . If the ethnography of meaning is not legitimated
> in primary care research, even though it is legitimated in anthropology,
> sociology, and social psychology, then meaning will not receive a scien-
> tifically appropriate assessment in primary care. (1983:543)

TRAINING RELATIONSHIP AND CLINICAL
ETHNOGRAPHY

Michael Balint (1957) was perhaps the most eloquent and persistent to argue that in biomedicine as in psychotherapy, the clinical

relationship is the basis for any intervention. Medical educators rarely make the further point that isomorphically, the attending/ resident and behavioral scientist/resident relationship is likewise the foundation of successful pedagogy. It is that relationship—and not exclusively the faculty member's specific factual expertise or skill—that determines whether it is emotionally safe or unsafe to bring up certain kinds of material for discussion (e.g., fears of failure, anger, clinical data outside the strictly biomedical model). And it is that relationship that determines whether clinically pertinent subjective material will be acknowledged or disavowed. It has long been the behavioral scientist coauthor's principal goal to foster a teaching atmosphere in which the student or resident (as well as the patient and family) feels emotionally safe, understood, and challenged.

The writers have collaborated since 1980, for the first two years in a behavioral scientist/resident relationship in a community-based residency training program, and until June 1984 as faculty members in the same department of family medicine. In the summer of 1984 the physician coauthor joined a partnership in a rural town in southern Oklahoma. During his residency the physician coauthor, interested in the role of subjectivity in medicine, had frequent discussions with the behavioral scientist coauthor on issues that are customarily regarded as interesting but extraneous in medical education: resident-staff interaction, the physician's own family, the influence of religion on doctor and patient alike, the influence of work setting on patient behavior and symptoms. Conversations about patient care invariably led to comparisons with one's own family situation, current or past.

During the residency training relationship between the two authors, the genogram and structural/functional family-assessment instruments had been routinely used and had aroused mostly perfunctory interest in the resident at the time. (In both of our experiences as family medicine teachers, most residents have regarded such instruments and techniques—whether used as tools of self-discovery or of family mapping—as a series of onerous forced steps and have tended to prepare them more grudgingly and compliantly than enthusiastically.) Discussions of "work"—occupation, livelihood, employment—were another matter, and tended to kindle lively discussion, especially among residents who felt chronically overworked and who had considerable empathy for patients from farming families for whom *work* was synonymous with *family*. Although the resident's parents were not farmers, they shared the widespread Great Plains family and culture pattern that values work above most other aspects of life. Moreover, for the resident as for his family, *work* was an acceptable topic of public discourse. The physician coauthor expressed interest in Oklahoma farming families, especially that of his in-laws, and we began to explore that interest during and subsequent to residency training. "Work" provided a natural bridge to "family," initially the family of his in-laws and eventually his family of origin.

The feel for systems, and thereby greater empathy for those systems of his patients, evolved on the physician coauthor's terms rather than being structured by the pedagogical instrument of the behavioral scientist. Ethnographically, the physician coauthor learned to shift back and forth between being "informant" or "subject" and "observer" or "researcher." It was, we believe, the behavioral scientist coauthor's willingness to respond serendipitously to the interest of the resident that fostered the resident's greater interest in the dynamics of his own family. Together we discovered that, beyond his family, among Great Plains "white" farming and domestic animal-husbanding families (e.g., wheat, corn, cattle, pigs) and their urban-living successors, there is a blur, if not a merger, between family or home and work or occupation (Bennett 1982; Stein 1983d) and a protective privacy about the intimacy of one's homelife. These facts commended a culturally tailored approach to teaching about families: e.g., a more indirect, understated, hinted rather than formally explicit, and gradualist approach not only with this resident but in general. To do otherwise was to be told that, one's teaching credentials notwithstanding, one was downright impolite.

The physician coauthor, his wife, and their families were from the northwest area of Oklahoma, often called the wheat belt. Moreover his father-in-law was himself a wheat farmer. The behavioral scientist coauthor had formulated some impressions, while teaching residents in a community-based program in that part of the state, about the relationship between the structure of farming families, values, the annual cycle of work activities, and the timing of the use of health care facilities (lowest utilization during harvest, even in the presence of grave illness). Having written a preliminary paper (1982a), he asked his colleague to take a look at it and comment on the plausibility of the interpretation. The physician-colleague shortly thereafter related the following incident at the father-in-law's home: "As I was reviewing the article on the 'annual cycle' over the weekend, the article gave me a picture of what I was seeing in my wife's family. I left the paper out in the living room, and returned only to find my father-in-law reading it, smiling and nodding his head as he went."

Shortly after that, we discussed the paper and the father-in-law's response to it. The family physician coauthor then used the paper as the point of departure to discuss his family's use of the health care system, and illustrated his points with case material from his own family. "Let me tell you about what recently happened with my father-in-law, because it is evidence for the point you are arguing"—namely, that wheat farmers and their families orient their lives to the cycle of the wheat crop (and of livestock), assuring that above all else they will be ready for the harvest (late June/early July) (Stein 1982a). Health care is planned so as to prepare for the harvest and in order not to interfere with it. The unfolding of that case is given later below.

The physician coauthor used the behavioral scientist's initial observations, combined with his own interests, to begin a closer investigation of the values, attitudes, beliefs, roles, and organization of his own family, and how that might affect not only their health behavior but his own behavior as a practitioner. First in the residency program, later as faculty colleagues, the coauthors met to discuss some recent family incident or emerging pattern, to test coauthors' notions about the relation between work, family, and health care in this family, and to examine how this might work in families of patients. Clinical work evoked a closer look at one's own family; issues raised by looking at one's own family prompted a closer look at families of patients.

The issue of timing and availability was critical here to convert a random event into a teaching moment (Stein 1983c). By taking an interest in his physician-colleague's interests, the behavioral science teacher piqued the physician's further interest in points the behavioral scientist was trying to convey. What the behavioral scientist is ready to teach must be constantly matched with what the physician resident or colleague is ready to learn. Moreover, if a picture is worth ten thousand words, then a good case or the airing of a personal issue with a trusted faculty member is worth ten thousand wordy lectures!

CASE 1: NO TIME FOR SURGERY

John Deer is a sixty-year-old white male who farms outside a small town in northern Oklahoma. He works fourteen to sixteen hours daily, and is upset when he is unable to work. His farming activities consist mainly of large-scale pork production and several sections of wheat land, which he and his son-in-law actively farm.

Over the last several years, John Deer has noticed that he was having increased difficulty with his right knee, especially when he bent down to work on feeders or when getting into a tractor cab. He visited several physicians to alleviate the pain. Although medication somewhat decreased the pain, when he would take it, Mr. Deer continued to have an intermittent effusion over the knee and experienced a marked loss in his range of motion. As the more active seasons (spring and early summer) in his farming operation came about, the knee pain became worse, but Mr. Deer protested to the family that during these periods he had little time to take care of it. He would wait until November, December, or January to have it checked, for winter was the time he felt that the farm needed the least amount of attention. For as long as possible, Mr. Deer postponed having anything major done about the knee, for fear that it would restrict his activities, and that he might come out of it worse than when he went in. It was observed by his family physician son-in-law [JMP] that: "For him not to have harvest is like a death notice." Mr. Deer relied on his family for medical advice and health care prior to and while utilizing medical facilities.

In October 1980, he consulted an orthopedic surgeon for evaluation in a city some thirty miles from home. He was told that he had severe degenerative arthritis of the knee. The orthopedic surgeon recommended a total knee prosthesis. Mr. Deer informed the physician that he would consider surgery, but needed time to think about it.

Mr. Deer returned home and asked the advice of his family physician son-in-law (at that time a second-year resident). The latter discussed with Mr. Deer the pros and cons of joint replacement, what he might expect in terms of outcome, and length of convalescence. Mr. Deer continued to have difficulty in making a decision.

At the suggestion of the family physician son-in-law, he obtained a "second opinion" from a physician at a well-known regional medical center—in its department of orthopedics—some one hundred miles from Mr. Deer's home. The second orthopedist concurred with the initial assessment and also recommended a total knee replacement.

Mr. Deer subsequently developed low back pain, which his original orthopedic surgeon felt was secondary to his gait (which had changed because of the pain he initially had in the right knee). The back pain persisted, motivating Mr. Deer to consult a local chiropractor, who had a reputation in the community of being able to improve resistant cases of back pain. Mr. Deer expected an instant cure (an assumption shared by many, that when one goes to the chiropractor for treatment, one will feel better immediately; treatment by physicians, on the other hand, takes time and its outcome is often uncertain). The chiropractor took a series of X rays, pointed out that indeed it was his back that was causing his pain, and that to operate would be futile, since it was the back that was the difficulty and would respond to "manipulation."

After the treatment by the chiropractor had failed to reduce his pain, Mr. Deer tarried another two months prior to making his decision to undergo the knee surgery. In February 1981 he decided to have the surgery done. The ingenious—and culturally appropriate—logic that the son-in-law employed to convince his father-in-law to undergo surgery in late winter was that, all things being equal, Mr. Deer should be mobile enough by late May to participate fully in the wheat harvest.

In early March 1981 a total knee prosthesis was performed. There were no intraoperative or postoperative complications. Mr. Deer was discharged to home in mid-March. At that time he had only sixty degrees range of motion in his right knee, and it was painful to ambulate. His orthopedic surgeon informed him that this restriction was entirely "within normal limits" and that he would gradually be able to increase his range of motion. His physical therapist, a daughter, worked consistently with him over the ensuing weeks to improve the range of motion. Mr. Deer was markedly dissatisfied with his progress. He was anxious, with the wheat harvest rapidly approaching, that he would be in no condition to oversee the harvesting of his crops.

The knee immobility also played a role in his investment in new equipment, specifically, a combine "with a cab large enough" to accommodate a leg in the extended position. This purchase would enable him to harvest his crops as he had done for forty years. Five months later, Mr. Deer had full range of motion of his right knee and contemplated having a prosthesis done on the left knee.

CASE 2: THE MIRACLE BACK CENTER

Mrs. Jane Case is a thirty-six-year-old white female who is the eldest daughter of John Deer [see case 1]. She is married and has two children, ages three and nine. She and her husband live and work on the family farm in northern Oklahoma.

She had been in fairly good health during her childhood and early adulthood. She had been noted in high school as having minimal scoliosis, but no intervention was advised at that time. Recently, Mrs. Case had had several episodes of bronchitis and pneumonia. Because of persistent fever and dehydration, she required hospitalization on one occasion, on which her scoliosis was once again noted. This resulted in a referral to the orthopedist in a nearby city. The orthopedist, on reevaluation, felt that the scoliosis had advanced to the point that it was predisposing Mrs. Case to the recurrent pneumonias.

In November 1983, she saw her orthopedic surgeon because she was having moderate to severe back pains. On examination it was noted that her scoliosis had advanced a total of thirty degrees in two years. She was advised that this was probably the etiology of her back pain and also played a role in her recurrent pneumonias. Further, the orthopedic surgeon advised that she consider surgical correction of the scoliosis and the placement of Harrington rods. He suggested several distant regional centers where this expensive and delicate surgery could be performed. He also gave her several names of patients who had had this surgery, for her to contact for further information.

Mrs. Case called a family physician brother-in-law [JMP] to ask for further information about scoliosis, the surgery, its implications and problems. She further asked if there were any physicians whom he would recommend for the surgery. She also expressed anxiety about the timing of the surgery and the distance from home that she would have to travel to get to a regional center. Because the recovery would involve eight to nine months in a body cast—during which time she would be limited in what she could do and would require assistance from other family members—timing was important, so as not to interfere with the work load on the family farm.

Since the family physician brother-in-law was teaching at one regional medical center, he was most familiar with the physicians on the medical school faculty who performed this surgery. Also, his experience with his orthopedic colleagues was very good, and he had no hesitation in recommending them highly. An appointment was made for Mrs. Case to be evaluated at the regional medical center.

In the meantime, Mrs. Case contacted several of the patients who had had previous scoliosis surgery. Many had good outcomes and were pleased with their surgeons. Mrs. Case personally visited one of these patients who had had a good outcome, and the patient was jubilant about the surgeon, the surgery, and the entire process. The only problem would be that this patient's surgeon practiced in another state, in a city 750 miles from Mrs. Case's home.

The family was having difficulty with the decision. They were giving Mrs. Case several messages: "You need to be careful about when you have the surgery, so as not to interfere with the farm work. It is quite a long way to the medical center, but of course you would want the most experienced surgeons doing the procedure." The Christmas holidays were also approaching and that would not be a good time for the surgery, spoiling the family togetherness of the holiday season. Ultimately, based on the recommendation of the satisfied patient, Mrs. Case cancelled the appointment made at the regional medical center, and arranged to be scheduled after the holidays to be evaluated for surgery at the medical center 750 miles from home. Her logic was that she was impressed by the patient's outcome and wanted a similar outcome for herself.

In January 1984, the surgery was performed. There were no intraoperative or postoperative complications. After a two-week hospital stay, Mrs. Case was released to convalesce at home. She tolerated the body cast without difficulty, although she continued to worry about what effect her relative disability would have on the farming activities of the family, especially as "harvest" would be accomplished without her.

Mrs. Case's position in the sibling order figures prominantly in her family's mixed feelings and messages toward her as she was deliberating whether, where, and when to have the surgery performed (e.g., have it/don't have it; leave for a remote medical center/don't leave us). Although the eldest of the three sisters, she has an older brother. Ideally, among Oklahoma farming families, the eldest son is groomed to inherit and manage the family farm. In this family, however, the eldest son while still a youngster, was scalded, to which his mother responded by protecting him and "hovering" over him. As a teenager, he sustained foot and back injuries from an automobile accident. While he now successfully holds a job and has married and has children, he was never reared to manage the farm. This role of successor fell early upon the future Mrs. Case, who lives with her husband and children on the family farm owned by John Deer.

In this family Mrs. Case was invested with the responsibilities and experienced the anxieties associated with being the eldest son. The family inadvertently pressured her to continue in her role at the same time that the disease process made that role increasingly difficult to uphold. In a sense, for her to have the surgery and not to have the surgery both posed threats to her and to her family's concern for their joint future.

CASE 3: FORTY YEARS OF SMOKE

These first two cases dealt with medical decision making in a Baptist Scotch-English wheat-farming family from northern Oklahoma. They readily reveal (*a*) the effect of family roles, priorities, values, and expectations on health care choices and timing; (*b*) the paramount value of work in the family structure; (*c*) the virtually indistinguishable domains of "family" and "work"; (*d*) the utilization of multiple health-care providers as part of the patient's and family's decision making strategy; (*e*) the influence of family and lay-referral networks on health care decisions and the management of illness episodes; and (*f*) the choice between locally based treatment and treatment at a regional health care center. It became evident to both writers that what physicians often regard as "background" in fact occupies the foreground of a family's health-related perceptions, decisions, and actions. These cases revealed the unseen context in which medical intervention occurs.

It may be objected that the case vignettes offered do not derive from the physician's family of origin, but from his in-laws. While that fact is true, the source of the data does not vitiate the validity of the method: (*a*) the physician's natal family, while not a farming family, comes from the same region and shares the dominant values, religion, roles, and health-related decision making patterns that obtain for the larger culture in which the family of in-laws is embedded; and (*b*) one is most capable of observing where one is most comfortable observing. One must begin somewhere, and the whole point is to begin. One may simply find one's in-laws to be a relatively safe point of departure.

Over time, the physician coauthor began to take an ethnographic look at his family of origin, with special emphasis on his father's cigarette smoking. The following case—and greater understanding of cigarette smokers—followed.

Mr. P is a sixty-two-year-old white male who works as a janitor for the public school system in a northern Oklahoma town. He is semi-retired from route sales for dairy products after becoming unable to keep up with the pace required secondary to his health. Mr. P had smoked one to two packs of cigarettes per day over the last forty years. He had made several attempts in the past to quit, mainly by abrupt cessation over a vacation with some success, stopping for two to three weeks at a time. A frequent Christmas gift, from his family, was the latest "gimmick" in smoking cessation. These usually ended up stored away after not being helpful in ending his smoking addiction.

In 1983 the patient began to notice increasing shortness of breath, chronic paroxsymal coughing episodes that would cause him to become somewhat confused, and a decrease in his work tolerance secondary to shortness of breath. He also noted that he was losing weight, although he had had no change in his diet or appetite. After this symptom pattern progressed for several months, he was continually harangued by his wife of forty years to go to his physician for an evaluation. He usually put her off by saying he "would get around to it" or "there is probably nothing they can do for me."

Over one holiday visit with his son, a family physician [JMP], Mr. P related his symptom complex and requested his son's impression, "What do you think I have?" He also expressed concern that he was having difficulty getting his work done because he was continually stopping to "catch my breath or coughing." [Once again the theme of "work" surfaced, helping the physician coauthor to understand the context in which a symptom is identified by an individual and/or family as meriting medical or other course of action.] The son explained to Mr. P that he had watched him progressively show the signs of Chronic Obstructive Pulmonary Disease (COPD) over the past several years. He explained that this had been his main impetus for getting Mr. P to quit smoking, since smoking only added to his disease process and symptom complex. Although stopping smoking would not cure his health problems, he continued to explain, it would slow its progression and enable him to continue to work.

On the family-physician son's recommendation Mr. P made an appointment with his personal family physician, an older family physician. During the visit Mr. P outlined his symptoms and underwent the exam without difficulty. The chest X ray and pulmonary function tests revealed the COPD. The remainder of the exam revealed significant elevation of the blood pressure, but otherwise no abnormalities were noted. Mr. P was started on antihypertensive medication and aminophylline and once again was advised to stop smoking.

Mr. P took his medication regularly, but made no attempt to decrease his smoking intake. He continued to feel weak and short of breath. He called his family physician son, asking if he ought to obtain a second opinion, as he was not feeling any better. When asked if he had stopped smoking, Mr. P sighed and stated "I can't." The son explained once again that the evaluation by Mr. P's physician had been appropriate, that he was on the appropriate medication, and that to obtain a second opinion would only increase medical costs and not provide additional information.

Several days later Mr. P called his son and asked if he would prescribe nicotine gum for him, as a coworker had utilized it recently to taper his tobacco intake. [As with Mrs. Case, here too the informal personal network, in addition to family members, proved to be important in understanding health decision making.] The son asked why Mr. P did not call his physician for a prescription. Mr. P answered, "He'd only give me a lecture and tell me to tough it out."

A prescription for the nicotine gum was phoned for Mr. P after instructions for its use were given over the phone. A follow-up phone call was made one week later, mainly to visit. The conversation drifted to the gum use, and Mr. P was ecstatic over his progress. He explained that it was the first time he had not felt "depressed" while quitting, and he was extremely encouraged by his progress. [This likewise marked the son's attempt to work *within* the father's framework.] Mr. P chewed the nicotine gum for approximately three weeks, completely discontinuing his smoking. His cough diminished considerably; he gained weight and began to lose some of his weakness. Although he persists in being short of breath with exertion, he can keep up with the duties of his current job.

Smoking cessation had always been a frustrating portion of the physician coauthor's practice. He was familiar with the frustration of being in a home where someone smoked. The health problems that he slowly saw his father develop, even when he was in high school, were one of the strongest motivators for him not to smoke, even when his peers attempted to pressure his participation. The physician's frustration in dealing with smoking cessation derived from his previous experience with his father. He found himself sitting in exam rooms with patients who smoked, lecturing them about why it is harmful and hearing them say "I need to quit," only to find them leaving the office parking lot smoking a cigarette. Since his father's success with the nicotine gum, the physician coauthor finds himself renewed in his attempt to help patients stop smoking and has gained some insight into how to work with smoking patients within the framework of their lives (e.g., with patients who highly value work, using this value as leverage to help "motivate" them). Finally, by developing greater empathy for patients and understanding symptoms within patients' personal, familial, and occupational contexts, he is more able to help patients and feels less the need to control their behavior.

DISCUSSION OF REGIONAL CULTURE

To conclude this section, we wish to go somewhat beyond what has been learned from inquiry into the physician coauthor's family of origin and in-law family. In the process of comparing these families with countless other Oklahoma "white" families seen clinically, and from numerous conversations with physicians and staffs about some family common denominators we thought we were seeing, we have willy-nilly encountered and subsequently formulated a regional cultural pattern (a "cultural areal ethos" [Devereux 1969]). From this understanding we have gained a greater sense of *how* to work clinically with patients and families in this region (Stein 1982b, 1984, 1985b, 1985c, 1987). For innumerable Great Plains families, issues that health professionals label as "mental health" and for which they would like to prescribe individual or family therapy (e.g., alcoholism, drug abuse, marital conflict, etc.) are instead labeled by families as associated with sin and family shame. The family-prescribed remedy for these chronic maladies is often a staunchly defended privacy and insularity. Family business is the business of no one else.

The regional prescription for depression is to put a smile on your face and go on with life. One rarely ventures to a psychiatrist or family therapist to talk about "family problems," lest the family's united front of well-being, harmony, and unity be shattered and the entire family be exposed to public criticism and ridicule. Patients too often fear that, should they disclose their weaknesses (which they construe as badness) to their physician (or to anyone else), they will receive the same stern judgment as their preacher metes out towering above them on the pulpit. Whenever a family member is diagnosed by the family as "crazy," the family rarely seeks treatment for this person. Instead, this person is hidden—often for decades—in the home, and kept even from church. "We take care of our own" is an oft-heard slogan, one that, among other functions that it serves, keeps family and would-be care giver at a considerable distance from each other.

The language of "faith" and "prayer" pervades discussion of human problems in this region. Likewise, the language of somaticization for patient and family alike is a way of saying that something is wrong with one's body without implicating self or family.

Family physicians, osteopathic physicians, and chiropractors flourish in this region, while to a considerable degree, except in the largest cities, the individual psychotherapies and family therapies tend to languish. This is not to say that therapy is impossible to conduct in this region, but that one must be prepared to work within the patient's and family's system of meanings and relationships rather than to impose one's own. We have found that patients feel comfortable in eventually discussing with family doctors and their consultants matters of sin, shame, and guilt that they would simply not bring to "mental health" specialists—and that the family doctor must learn to go slow at the patient's and family's pace. Otherwise the family will feel exposed or condemned and abruptly terminate treatment. In our own clinical work, we have often let patients and their families be our own teachers and guides into how and when we may offer intervention.

We have learned the importance—for patients, families, and ourselves alike—of friendliness, openness, indirectness, hints rather than direct confrontations or orders, patience, understatement, and avoidance of any threat that can be construed as a violation of the patient's or family's independence. When family pride, and fear of the exposure of secrets, can be honored, when family members can feel safe, then secrets that have often been kept for generations will be disclosed. But we have learned that the family physician must give the family plenty of time over time (which is why the family medicine ideal of "continuity of care" especially suits this patient population). And we have learned that one must not be too eager or rigid about assembling "the whole family" for family counseling or therapy. Often the only occasion on which the family is willing to convene with the doctor is while a family member is in the hospital— and at such times, the family is often eager to meet together with the doctor, but only in the hospital. At other times, the family doctor can make a "family intervention" through whomever is present in the clinic. None of this "cultural tailoring" of medical practice would have been a priori self-evident without the ethnography we have described in this section.

CONCLUSION AND IMPLICATIONS FOR MEDICAL TRAINING

In this chapter we have argued that the teacher-resident relationship, together with the larger context in which that teaching and supervision occurs (clinic, hospital, etc.), is inseparable from the didactic content, and affects how and what one is able to teach. How one teaches is, in this framework, closely guided by how the residents best learn. It requires in the teacher an enormous flexibility, tolerance for anxiety, and capacity for almost continuous reframing; the rewards—which come on the students' and residents' own time, not the teacher's schedule—are exhilarating. This chapter described one such successful odyssey.

This chapter concludes that the collaborative process that utilized the ethnographic style is inseparable from the product. One cannot truly speak of the teaching method distinct from the relationship, for the relationship is itself the method. Moreover, the history of a subject turns out to be the history of a particular teacher/resident and faculty colleague relationship. Rather than this being an occasion for despair—since serendipity is never precisely replicated elsewhere—it is, in fact, a pedagogical, scientific, and clinical opportunity. By fostering similar open-ended teaching relationships in family medicine, we may perhaps foster in ourselves and in others the scientific spirit of open-ended inquiry, curiosity, surprise, and serendipitous insight.

The ethnographic approach to clinical training bears some comment. It is one whose rigor lies in its very tolerance for ambiguity, its cultivation of open-endedness, and its potential for discovery and novelty. It is intended to complement and test culturally official and standardized pedagogical methods that are based upon predetermined behavioral objectives, performance criteria, and conceptual/technical outcomes. Through it, the physician becomes attentive—on his or her own terms, through the guidance of the teacher—to matters usually regarded as outside or peripheral to the purview of medical diagnosis and treatment.

With this approach, the student and resident learn that they are always working within a complex interlacing of contexts, and begin to take the time—over time—to elicit those contexts and to learn to work within them. Many residents discover, independent of teacher inculcation (read: nagging), that they stand a better chance of influencing medical outcomes by working within rather than against family systems and their metaphors. They likewise learn, as was evidenced in this chapter, what metaphors serve as the royal road to the family ("work") and which are taboo, at least for a time. And they come to accept, more from conviction than coercion, that family relationships and meanings make a difference in the management of an illness episode.

We have been told by family practice residents countless times over the years that they wish to be known as "doctors"—not so much in the etymological sense of "teacher" as in the cultural sense of "doer," master and conqueror of "real disease"—and they often bristle when called "therapists," "counselors," and the like. Behavioral science must, to be even remotely acceptable, approach family medicine residents on their "home ground." It should come as no surprise that residents who find their lived personal world taken seriously, with an effort made to work within that world, come to take the experienced and contextual world of their patients and patients' families and communities more seriously and to make greater effort to work within their world as well. We must specify the kind of learning this is, for it is not so much didactically inculcated as lived; the verbalization of the process comes late if at all. The dynamic is more of empathy and identification than of explicit role modeling or of inculcation of technique. Any outcome studies of this method must be congruent with this process. We have had a number of medical students and residents who have openly rejected this approach to teaching and patient care, only to tell us months or years later that it had taken root and that there was "something" to it after all. There is more to clinical learning than immediacy of recall.

A premise of this ethnographically informed training approach is that if the timing and appositeness of an intervention—biomedical, psychiatric, family therapy, etc.—together with the quality of the relationship upon which the intervention lasts, hold the key to therapy, these same dynamics hold the key to effective clinical teaching. Although the authors have clear content and topics in mind, these tend to unfold as they become clinically pertinent rather than being offered in a prestructured sequence. Stated differently, *the ethnographic model of family medicine training is relationship-and-context centered rather than exclusively teacher-and-topic centered.* The behavioral science material is thus less imposed by the authors than offered at clinically or developmentally key points in residents' experiences (Stein and Grant 1986).

The resident's readiness for the new material is a crucial issue. At its best the method has the effect of feeling as if the resident is discovering or inventing contextual assessment and intervention instead of having it intrusively (untimely) given or "packaged" (a word current in educational circles today). The new content thus becomes "theirs" as well as "ours," and tends to be experienced more in the spirit of play than of persecutory control (Winnicott

1967). The educational method we advocate is designed more to *help* the resident think, perceive, feel, and plan than to *mold or control* the resident's behavior (deMause 1974).

The ethnographic approach to clinical teaching and residency training takes an admittedly marked departure from traditional medical (and cultural) pedagogy that is exclusively lineal, sequential, future-oriented, and whose methods rely largely upon the inculcation of the "correct" way to think. The proposed approach does not entirely impugn this cultural convention, but suggests that such a convention, by itself, ends up being an orthodoxy that may in turn prevent the medical student or resident from discovering anything that departs from such a closed scheme. Cultural materials such as genograms, family circles, and functional/structural family assessments are used as "levers" (Devereux 1969), as potentially useful means to the clinical end—but such means are discardable when the resident and instructor together discover better means to that end. For instance, while we might discuss various instruments of family assessment, we also begin to recognize and point out their culture-boundedness, e.g., in the implicit conviction that "normal" is in the middle, balanced, never extreme (How would Galileo fare?), that normality can be located on a straight line. Such instruments can be used to illustrate culture rather than blindly to inculcate it.

The ethnographic approach *helps* residents to learn (the impetus being from within as much as from without) to a greater extent than it *socializes* residents concerning what to learn (see deMause [1974] for a psychohistorical approach to this distinction). The teacher functions more as a guide than a drillmaster. This is not to say that the teacher does not teach, does not come highly prepared with concepts and skills, but that the teacher is also prepared to respond to the resident's promptings, to follow the resident's lead *in order to* convey those concepts and skills with the maximum likelihood that they will be learned. The teacher in this scheme does the utmost to include the residents' world in how and when those concepts and skills are presented.

In this chapter we have argued that the clinical use of the ethnographic method as a training tool of family medicine teaching, research, and patient care is both methodologically sound and practical. It helps us to flesh out the data we seek, that is, the lived reality of people in sickness, health, and treatment. Truth is to be found in the courage of ambiguity and the painstaking pursuit of details, not in inculcating the compulsive certitude of broad brushstrokes that make fact the handmaiden of belief.

Our methods must be true to our subject matter. As Whitehead said, "a one-sided formulation may be true, but may have the effect of a lie by its distortion of emphasis" (1960:123). Whether we like it or not, there is no way to read others' minds or lives or families. To pursue what Maranhão wryly calls "snapshot anthropology" (1984:270) as if it offered accurate portraits of people's lives in sickness and health is to confuse the pursuit of convenience with the nature of the subject we are trying to comprehend. There exist no shortcuts in data gathering and data interpretation that do not falsify the elusive and complex reality we are trying to chronicle and explain—and then treat. Indeed, the quest for such shortcuts are ipso facto quests for institutionalized defenses that protect us from the anxiety that more intensive and extensive inquiry might evoke. We ultimately know that which we do not seek to know. And while this is understandable as a very human response, it is not given us as teachers or practitioners or scientists to indulge it—it is our responsibility to identify and understand it instead.

As the many controversies within anthropology over cultural interpretation attest (e.g., the recent one over Margaret Mead's interpretation of adolescence in Samoa), the use of the ethnographic method does not by itself guarantee that one will not use the method for defensive purposes against self-knowledge and insight into those whom one is studying. Observation and interpretation are always acts of selection; the question is whether one is aware of the selection, of the meaning of that selection, and thereby has the capacity to modify the process of selection. The corrective that will enhance clinical observation is for clinical teacher and resident alike to become more self-observant.

To one knowledgeable in the history of medicine, the *naturalistic* approach to the psychosocial and historical realm would be congruent with, if not simply an extension of, the inquisitive naturalism we associate in biomedicine with such luminaries as Hippocrates, Leonardo da Vinci, Sir William Harvey, Sir Alexander Fleming, Louis Pasteur, and Robert Koch (see Kuzel 1986). The practice of medicine in the United States is being increasingly subjected to simplification and regimentation of clinical thought, standardization, centralized outside control, mechanization, and a minimalist philosophy of responsibility (Kormos 1984; Stein and Hill 1984; Stephens 1984a, 1984b, 1984c). Yet the sound exercise of clinical judgment depends upon context-embedded thinking and planning on the part of the clinician. It is indispensable to good patient care irrespective of the official political-medical climate. The use of the ethnographic method to describe and explain the family dynamics of health behavior—together with the group dynamics of medical practice itself—will be a valuable tool for practitioners, teachers, and researchers who wish to help physicians (indeed, practitioners) of all specialties and disciplines to think and practice contextually.

REFERENCES

Alexander, L. 1979. Clinical anthropology: Morals and methods. *Medical Anthropology* 3:61–107.

Balint, M. 1957. *The doctor, his patient, and the illness.* New York: International Universities Press.

Bennett, J. W. 1982. *Of time and the enterprise: North American family farm management in a context of resource marginality.* Minneapolis: University of Minnesota Press.

Bowen, M. 1978. *Family therapy in clinical practice.* New York: Jason Aronson.

Cromwell, R., D. Fournier, and D. Kvebaek. 1980. *The Kvebaek family sculpture technique: A diagnostic and research tool in family therapy.* Jonesboro, Tenn.: Pilgrimage.

DeMause, L., ed. 1974. *The history of childhood.* New York: Psychohistory Press.

Devereux, G. 1969. *Reality and dream: Psychotherapy of a Plains Indian.* New York: New York University Press (orig. 1951).

Geertz, C. 1973. *The interpretation of cultures: Selected essays.* New York: Basic Books.

Kleinman, A. 1983. The cultural meanings and social uses of illness: A role for medical anthropology and clinically oriented social science in the development of primary care theory and research. *The Journal of Family Practice* 16(3):539–45.

Kormos, H. R. 1984. The industrialization of medicine. In *Advances in medical social sciences,* vol. 2, edited by J. L. Ruffini, 323–39. New York: Gordon and Breach Science Pubs.

Kuzel, A. J. 1986. Naturalistic inquiry: An appropriate model for family medicine. *Family Medicine* 18(6):369–74.

La Barre, W. 1978. The clinic and the field. In *The making of psychological anthropology,* edited by G. D. Spindler, 258–99. Berkeley and Los Angeles: University of California Press.

Maranhão, T. 1984. Family therapy and anthropology. *Culture, Medicine and Psychiatry* 8:255–79.

Olson, D. H., H. I. McCubbin, H. Barnes, A. Larsen, M. Muzen, and M. Wilson. 1982. *Family inventories.* St. Paul: Department of Family Social Science, University of Minnesota.

Pendagast, E. G., and C. O. Sherman. 1977. A guide to the genogram family systems training. *The Family* 5(1):3–14.

Schwartzman, H. B., A. W. Kneifel, L. Barbera-Stein, and E. Gaviria. 1984.

Children, families, and mental health service organizations: Cultures in conflict. *Human Organization* 43(4):297–306.

Schwartzman, J., ed. 1985. *Families and other systems: The macrosystemic context of family therapy.* New York: Guilford Press.

Spiro, M. E. 1982. *Buddhism and society: A great tradition and its Burmese vicissitudes,* 2d expanded edition. Berkeley and Los Angeles: University of California Press.

Stein, H. F. 1982a. The annual cycle and the cultural nexus of health care behavior among Oklahoma wheat farming families. *Culture, Medicine and Psychiatry* 6(1):81–99.

———. 1982b. The ethnographic mode of teaching clinical behavioral science. In *Clinically applied anthropology: Anthropologists in health science settings,* edited by N. Chrisman and T. Maretzki, 61–82. Boston: D. Reidel.

———. 1982c. Physician-patient transaction through the analysis of countertransference: A study in role relationship and unconscious meaning. *Medical Anthropology* 6(3):165–82.

———. 1983a. The case study method as a means of teaching significant context in family medicine. *Family Medicine* 15(5):163–67.

———. 1983b. The influence of counter-transference upon the clinical relationship and decision-making. *Continuing Education for the Family Physician* 18(7):625–30.

———. 1983c. Review essay—Investing psyche and capital: Farming and its hidden meanings. Review of *Of time and the enterprise: North American family farm management in a context of resource marginality,* by J. W. Bennett. *The Journal of Psychoanalytic Anthropology* 6(1):91–98.

———. 1983d. The "teaching moment." *Family Medicine* 15(5):191–92.

———. 1984. Sittin' tight and bustin' loose: Contradiction and conflict in Midwestern masculinity and the psychohistory of America. *The Journal of Psychohistory* 11(4):501–12.

———. 1985a. *The psychodynamics of medical practice: Unconscious factors in patient care.* Berkeley and Los Angeles: University of California Press.

———. 1985b. Therapist and family values in cultural context. *Counseling and Values* 30(1):35–46.

———. 1985c. Values and family therapy. In *Families and other systems: The macrosystemic context of family therapy,* edited by J. Schwartzman, 201–43. New York: Guilford Press.

———. 1987. Farmer and cowboy: The duality of the Midwestern male ethos—A study in ethnicity, regionalism, and national identity. In *From metaphor to meaning: Papers in psychoanalytic anthropology,* vol. 2 of the Series in Ethnicity, Medicine, and Psychoanalysis, by H. F. Stein and M. Apprey, 178–227. Charlottesville: University Press of Virginia.

Stein, H. F., and M. Apprey. 1985. *Context and dynamics in clinical knowledge,* vol. 1 of the Series in Ethnicity, Medicine, and Psychoanalysis. Charlottesville: The University Press of Virginia.

Stein, H. F., and W. D. Grant. 1986. *Behavioral science in family medicine: A program for second and third year family medicine residents.* Kansas City: The Society of Teachers of Family Medicine.

Stein, H. F., and R. F. Hill. 1984. American medicine and the enchanted machine. *Continuing Education for the Family Physician* 19(8):428–30.

Stephens, G. G. 1984a. Five aspects of the healer. *Continuing Education for the Family Physician* 19(12):663–66.

——. 1984b. The medical supermarket: Futuristic or decadent? *Continuing Education for the Family Physician* 19(5):243, 245.

——. 1984c. The medical supermarket: Futuristic or decadent? part 2. *Continuing Education for the Family Physician* 19(11):600–610.

Whitehead, A. N. 1960. *Religion in the making.* Cleveland and New York: Meridian (orig., 1926).

Winnicott, D. W. 1967. The location of cultural experience. *International Journal of Psychoanalysis* 48:368–72.

Conclusions:
Toward an
Ethnographic-Psychoanalytic Paradigm
of Clinical Stories

MAURICE APPREY AND HOWARD F. STEIN

To help people to be able to tell their own stories, and to work with and within those stories—tales that usually are masked by yet other, more acceptable, conventional stories—is the core therapeutic function. This is so irrespective of how a malady is culturally labeled: biomedical disease, mental illness, family dysfunction, psychopathology, deviance, social problem, and so forth. Numerous variations on this theme and premise have been presented throughout the book.

Chapters in part I described the process and the outcome of clinical relationships in which the narrating of the story is at once diagnostic and part of the healing itself. Listening "with the third ear," that of the clinician's unconscious, as Theodor Reik (1948) wonderfully called it, is the reciprocal dynamic that fosters the unfolding of the patient's or family's inner drama. The range of clinical material or "entities"—spinal cord injury, witchcraft, anorexia nervosa, and a multitude of physical disabilities—has illustrated the central theme that it is the often widely shared intrapsychic story that gives meaning to the expression of the pathology, if not to the "symptom choice" itself.

The tendency in many modern therapeutic and biomedical schools of thought to isolate and decontextualize symptoms and to define pathology narrowly only substitutes anxiety-alleviating diagnostic and treatment narratives for the deeper, more painful ones that the clinician "helps" patient and family alike not to have to hear. The chapters in part I portrayed the depth, breadth, and often bewildering complexity of symptoms and their meanings as far more the rule than the much wished-for exception in all clinical practice. "You are a servant of the process," is a favorite motto of psychoanalyst James Masterson (1983)—a process that assists patients and families in telling and facing their own stories.

That process of knowing—of knowing anything—is always presided over by anxiety. There ever lurks the danger that one will notice or observe the wrong thing, ask the wrong questions, juxtapose ideas that do not "rightfully" belong together. Anxiety signals to us when we approach or violate the boundary of the knowable. This is not only true of patients and families in need of a healer's help but of healers and their teachers as well. The limitations on what one may know limit, if not constrict, how one may truly be helpful toward those in one's clinical care. Knowing is such a precarious issue that one requires a method, a road map as it were, to see one's way through a multitude of resistances: the practitioner's own, the patient's own, that of the medical or therapeutic establishment, the larger culture it serves, and the very complexity of pathological formation and treatment. The chapters in part II have offered a psychoanalytically oriented ethnographic method in clinical education and supervision, an approach that focuses on understanding and working within the personal history of the individual clinician trainee and the official and unofficial stories that give coherence to clinical institutions.

The method discussed in the final four chapters paralleled exactly that more explicitly clinical method discussed earlier in terms of patient care. Chapters in part I have documented the resistance patients and their families (and persons in their wider contexts) bring to recognizing the intrapsychic story, and the therapeutic process by which the story is allowed to emerge. Chapters in part II similarly examined the contribution of the individual clinician's unconscious, family-of-origin experience, and larger institutional and culture ethos to resistance to clinical knowing, and likewise discuss a training context-sensitive method whereby access to his/her own intrapsychic story—and thereby to that of his/her patients or clients—is fostered. The very existence of these chapters challenges a much cherished illusion that practitioners and patients alike tenaciously hold: that clinicians and clients are essentially dissimilar in psychological makeup, that a doctor is not a patient. By contrast, only to the degree that we can acknowledge and "own" and comprehend our own patienthood can we truly help others.

Throughout this book we have argued, and illustrated, not only that the story behind the story completes the initial account, but that the latent story is a part of the manifest one. From the viewpoint of the topographical or spatial organizational metaphor of the mind, the manifest and latent are separate and distinct. However, from the viewpoint of time, they are continuous, synchronous. The same story appears at different levels at different times during clinical training or in clinical relationships. The manifest story is in conventional cultural language; the latent tale in unconventional language. For the careful listener, teacher, or clinician, the latent is often part of the flow of the manifest, its voice only waiting to be heard. The manifest is, as it were, grafted upon the latent one, receiving its nourishment from the very roots whose influence it tries to hide. We have proposed that a depth psychology–informed ethnographic approach is a fruitful method for obtaining and treating the story behind the story: of clinicians, students, teachers, patients, and families alike.

It is not always possible for the administrator, clinician, or clinical teacher to apply the methods of depth psychology to the human drama that he or she faces in his or her work and to explore extensively dynamic issues of the unconscious that may be involved. At the very least it is one's responsibility to employ a variation of psychoanalytic methods of observation in order to understand the human dramas that lie behind difficulties faced by students, interns, resident, staff, and faculty.

Medical students and professionals come from all walks of life, different cultures and races, all sorts of colleges, and all kinds of religious backgrounds. If we want to be effective, we must be able to use psychological understanding without alienating them.

What might this variation of psychoanalytic observation be? We take the position that academic, residency, or clinical difficulties constitute a drama in which the student, apprentice clinician, or practitioner is at the center of a number of events that have a personal meaning for him or her. Following Politzer (1967), we call these precipitated dramas original "first person dramas," seeing in them psychological facts that are original insofar as they were created by the student or resident or practitioner himself or herself, wittingly, or unwittingly, to solve a particular problem or perceived catastrophe. These original human dramas follow a plan, and are located where the student is. The current surroundings of the student are woven into them. In other words, the medical school, internship, or residency environment is the stage on which the drama is being played out, but it is not the sole determinant of the drama.

As psychoanalyst/administrator (Apprey) and anthropologist/ teacher/clinical supervisor (Stein), we must take into account the psychological-familial-cultural issues that are outside the student's or resident's sphere of consciousness, and help the student or resident to bring to the surface and transcend the maladaptive responses that seem destined to destroy an otherwise promising career through academic failure, or that plague clinical work.

In our teaching and administrative roles, we expect to see unconscious repetitions in this setting, but we do not interpret them as such, or at least initially we stay at the student or resident's level of the story line. We see continuity and symmetry between unconscious and conscious psychological issues, and make decisions with or for students and residents as necessary, without verbalizing the linking interpretations involved or clarifying deep genetic-developmental manifestations. Both language and gesture help to reveal the student's or resident's story: the former disclosing intentions, the latter indicating how these intentions come to life. Intentions strongly modify the dramas of daily life, and disclose their purposes.

To recapitulate the argument of this book, let us illustrate how intentions insert themselves into the lives of some students in ways that reveal their original personal stories. We present these vignettes along a spectrum, at one end of which the presenting difficulties are largely situational and at the other end of which they bear the symbolic burden of a lifetime. The case material is drawn from the psychoanalyst/administrator's (Apprey's) clinical notes.

VIGNETTE 1: THINGS ARE WHAT THEY SEEM

This first vignette describes the kind of student who approaches the Student Affairs Dean with a fairly circumscribed problem.

Adam's problem was that he had been served with a summons to respond to a paternity suit while he was in the middle of an anatomy examination. As dramatic as this kind of problem may seem, it is administratively quite easy to solve. The examination can be postponed, and subsequent meetings with the student can provide appropriate support. Other onetime, circumscribed problems might be the need to make funeral arrangements for a close relative, or the serious illness of the next of kin that necessitates returning home.

VIGNETTES 2 AND 3: THINGS ARE MORE THAN THEY SEEM

Sometimes, however, what seems to be a onetime, circumscribed problem can be deceptively complicated. A student or resident's problem may in fact be a mirror image of a prior one, or a subtle (or blatant) transformation of a prior one.

Abe, for instance, asked that his examination be rescheduled because his preparation for it had been seriously compromised by his being in the middle of getting a divorce. His examination was rescheduled, but during the next semester he again asked for rescheduling, this time for a different reason—the need to spend so much time with an alcoholic roommate that he was not able to prepare himself.

In this kind of situation appropriate counseling may be offered to prevent further repetition of this behavior once the human drama underlying the student's difficulties has been grasped.

To cite another brief example from Dr. Apprey,

although *Cain* had had a relatively problem-free first year, he failed the first examination in his second, and his performance in other courses was unsatisfactory. Toward the end of the year I learned by accident that he planned to get married during the summer following his second year. How, in a period of eight weeks, was he to negotiate a reexamination, perhaps a remedial summer course in another university, and a marriage? I called Cain to my office to ask why he planned what was so evidently a self-destructive course of action. Reluctantly Cain explained that his bride-to-be was already pregnant, and they did not want to have a baby out of wedlock. I heard also that her parents had come from the West Coast to urge him to marry her without delay, lest the promising young doctor fall into the hands of another woman.

Knowing what a destructive path Cain had devised, I invited him to bring his girlfriend for a breakfast meeting with me. Meeting her, I felt that she was unaware of what was happening in Cain's life in medical school, and that were she to become aware, she might not go through with the scheduled marriage. I created a background of safety that would allow him to tell her what was happening to him in medical school, and in her case the kind of life she was proposing to share. They had much to learn from one another, as it turned out, and they resolved to postpone their marriage.

Cain did not, however, want me to go away thinking that his decision to marry or to father a child was heedless. He went on to explain that while playing baseball a year earlier he had hurt his scrotum, and his physician had said that he had a low sperm count. Fearing that he would be unable to father a child, he had coaxed his reluctant girlfriend to test whether this were true or not. He had then proved himself; the girl was pregnant. With appropriate guidance, he is now well on his way to becoming a doctor.

Questions about the student's judgment arise in this type of situation, but it is not until the human drama underlying the manifestation of apparently poor judgment is seen that the drive to reenact or repeat a self-destructive series of original psychological events discloses itself. Offering or providing structure becomes part of caring as well as part of understanding how to help the student triumph over the original psychological events he or she is driven to replay.

This type of situation has problems that repeat themselves in a new edition or facsimile. They tend to have pervasive consequences that make one question the character or judgment of the student until the human drama has been carefully identified.

VIGNETTE 4: REPETITION OF A LONG HISTORY
OF TRAUMA

A different kind of repetition occurs here. It is predictable, and its consequences can be controlled. In this vignette of Dr. Apprey,

Naomi complained that a fellow student had stolen the homework she had finished. A week later she reported that someone had taken her purse—which she later found without its contents. Days later, her purse was again missing, and this time she was dealing with the loss of several hundred dollars. She called me at home at two o'clock in the morning to announce that she was going home, away from the medical school. I told her that I was not going to see her at that hour, but would discuss things with her the following morning, if she would stay that long. She insisted that her brother would be driving here to take her home.

When I went to her dormitory at nine o'clock the following morning as we had agreed, there she sat, sobbing heavily. There was something very striking about her tears, which seemed to me the tears of mourning rather than those evoked by a money loss. I asked if she had talked to her mother, and she replied that she had not because her mother was handicapped and must not be troubled. When I asked if she had spoken to her father, she replied that he was dead. She was surprised at my asking when he had died, but told me that he had died eight years earlier. When I asked the date of his death, she replied July 14. July 14 was today! With a little more detail to go on, I surmised that we were dealing with an anniversary reaction with anticipatory grief.

This story illustrates that an administrator, clinician, or teacher who has been able to anticipate the presence of this complicated kind of mourning can avert or control difficulties that it can cause. Psychotherapy is recommended in such cases. However, one must be alert to the subtle footprints of the unconscious story in the midst of the most conventional-appearing scene.

VIGNETTE 5: THE CURRENT STORY AS PART OF A
LIFETIME NARRATIVE

Here an invariant personal fantasy is invariably woven into the enactment of the story. For instance, students who are studying medicine for unsublimated reasons produce huge challenges. The Student Affairs Dean coauthor, Dr. Apprey, personally treated some of these students in three-, four-, or five-times weekly sessions of psychoanalysis. Here, however, he will describe the case of one who has not as yet received treatment and who failed to make the grades he needed to stay in medical school. His was a consultation arranged by the dean of a major London teaching hospital with whom Dr. Apprey worked on anorexia nervosa research and who knew of his interest in the psychological issues that impede learning.

Peter came to see me for a consultation. He had been failing in his first two years of medical school, and a faculty committee had asked him to leave. He disagreed with the committee's decision inasmuch as until then he had done everything asked by the dean's office, taking psychological tests, remedial workshops, educational assessments, etc. He claimed that the findings were inconclusive, although one assessor had noted that he was obsessed over the answers before finally writing down an incorrect reply. He claimed that he actually knew the substance of the basic sciences quite well, and reported that a professor had taken him home for one weekend to tutor and quiz him. Usually after three hours of this teaching and quizzing there was no doubt in the mind of either man that he knew the answers to the same questions he had answered incorrectly in written examinations.

Peter turned to me because he wished for me to be his advocate. He thought that as an analyst I might be able to pick up unconscious material from him that could help him plead his case with the dean of the medical school, who had the power to reinstate him.

He was angry that the dean had taken what he considered a long time to reply to requests for his intervention. He was even more angry that a former dean of student affairs had failed to save him from the decisions of the medical school faculty. Why couldn't that dean have saved him? After all, he had saved another student who had found himself in a like situation. Peter could not believe that a dean could only make recommendations about how to stay out of academic trouble but lacked the executive power to stave off the ire of the medical school faculty.

I asked him to tell me about himself in any way and any order that suited him. He said he was one of two siblings, born years after the first "because there was something wrong with my mother's womb for a long time, and just when they were about to operate (hysterectomy) I came along." He said that his parents had treated him well; they loved him. "My mother had *a second chance. My father, too, had a second chance* [emphasis added, M.A.]; he was the only man to have kept his place at Sandhurst after failing a course." He explained that since he had come from the British highlands, his father had had an education that fell short of preparing him in some academic areas for Sandhurst, and that the authorities there had understood this. "Why won't the medical school give me *a second chance?*" [emphasis added, M.A.], he demanded.

I learned in an hour-long interview that this student had failed to understand (1) the seriousness of his academic deficiencies; (2) the position of the student affairs dean who had been guiding him; (3) that second chances are not always available and that, in fact, the faculty could well have taken action against him much earlier; (4) that he had been overvalued by his family because of the circumstances of his birth; and (5) that they had spared him from experiencing anxiety, which is something that makes reasonable people sufficiently intelligent to anticipate and avoid danger.

It was evident that being dismissed had brought him massive narcissistic injury—and shame. He thought it beneath him to be placed in such a situation.

I recommended that he consult a nationally known educational specialist of my acquaintance so she could test him, and correct what seemed to her to be the problem. If, after correcting or even partly removing the "educational obstacles" in his path, he and the specialist agreed that he could continue, the medical school administration would entertain an application for his readmission.

I did not articulate a second recommendation that I would convey were he readmitted: that he consider intensive psychotherapy or psychoanalysis. I would do whatever else I could to effect his retention and subsequent graduation since I had reason to believe in his great ability to give care to others. Clearly, he would have to work on the narcissism that was keeping him from accepting help from others.

He promised to consult the educational specialist, and did get in touch with her. *But he talked her out of intervening.* Consequently, he is no longer in medical school.

Here, a whole lifetime and family ethos of entitlement crystallize around and into the issue of academic performance in medical school (see Volkan and Rodgers 1988). The latter is thus at once a part of the story and a symptom of the unconscious story that, at least for now, is not pursued.

These vignettes represent a spectrum or continuum of stories enacted, told, or dramatized by medical students in situations of learning, students, who, for psychological or other reasons, could not achieve their academic ends without intervention. We are not here referring to students who are weak academically, but to those who, having entered the professional school with better than average credentials, baffled administrators and teachers as to why they were failing or having unanticipated difficulty with their work.

Just as there are stories behind patients' and families' afflictions, there are also stories behind a medical student's academic problem or behind an intern's or resident's clinical problem (e.g., the proverbial "difficult patient"). Such stories can conceal some aspects of the problem while revealing others through enactments, new editions of the original personal story, or forms of acting out that are tantamount to remembering in action. This book has sought to bring to the forefront of clinical thinking, teaching, decision making, and clinical work the complex, sinuous texture of clinicians' and patients' stories, and the often fateful consequences of their interplay in clinical relationships, assessment, treatment, and outcome.

REFERENCES

Masterson, J. 1983. *Countertransference and psychotherapeutic technique.* New York: Brunner/Mazel.

Politzer, G. 1967. *Critique des fondements de la Psychologie.* Paris: Presses Universitaires de France.

Reik, T. 1948. *Listening with the third ear: The inner experience of a psychoanalyst.* New York: Farrar, Straus.

Volkan, V. D., and T. C. Rodgers, eds. 1988. *Attitudes of entitlement.* Charlottesville: University Press of Virginia.

A Note about the Authors

MAURICE APPREY, PH.D. (Member, Association of Child Psychotherapists, England), is a London-trained child analyst. He is Director of the Division of Ethnic Studies, a member of the Division of Psychoanalytic Studies, and Associate Professor in the Department of Behavioral Medicine and Psychiatry, University of Virginia School of Medicine, Charlottesville, Virginia.

MARY MARGARET KELLY, PH.D., is a faculty member of the Medical College of Virginia and Staff Psychologist, Virginia Treatment Center for Children, both in Richmond, Virginia.

JAMES MICHAEL PONTIOUS, M.D., is Medical Director, Garfield County Medical Society Family Practice Residency Program (University of Oklahoma), Enid, Oklahoma.

LARRY ROEDIGER, P.A.-C, M.P.H., received his training in occupational medicine through the University of Oklahoma College of Public Health and the Physician's Associate Program's graduate curriculum in Oklahoma City. He is Human Resources Manager at CLR Manufacturing Incorporated at Winston-Salem, North Carolina.

HOWARD F. STEIN, PH.D., a psychoanalytic anthropologist, is Professor in the Department of Family Medicine at the University of Oklahoma Health Sciences Center, Oklahoma City, Oklahoma, where he is coordinator of Intern and Resident Balint Seminars. He coordinates the behavioral sciences curriculum at the Enid Family Medicine Clinic residency training program. He edited *The Journal of Psychoanalytic Anthropology* from 1980 to 1988.

G. GAYLE STEPHENS, M.D., a family physician, is former chairman of the Department of Family Medicine, University of Alabama School of Medicine, Birmingham, Alabama. Former President of the Society of Teachers of Family Medicine, he is author of *The Intellectual Basis of Family Medicine,* and Associate Editor of the *Journal of the American Board of Family Practice.*

PAUL E. TIETZE, M.D., a family physician, is Associate Residency Director, Tuscaloosa Family Practice Residency Program, University of Alabama School of Medicine, Tuscaloosa, Alabama.

Index